Introdu

As a seasoned doctor with decades of experience in understanding the complexities of human health, one thing I have learned is that there is one organ often overlooked, yet it plays an indispensable role in keeping our body functioning—our liver. Whether you are young or old, healthy or battling certain conditions, liver health is something that everyone should prioritize, and here's why.

The liver is a silent hero in our body. It works relentlessly every day to detoxify the body, regulate hormones, store essential vitamins and minerals, produce bile for digestion, and manage blood sugar levels. Despite its immense importance, it is easy to forget about it until something goes wrong. This oversight can lead to liver dysfunction, a condition that can develop slowly, without symptoms at first, but eventually wreak havoc on your overall health.

I have dedicated my career to understanding liver disease and helping my patients avoid its devastating consequences. This book will provide you with the knowledge you need to protect your liver, enhance its function, and understand the warning signs that your liver may need attention. It's time to start treating your liver with the care and respect it deserves.

Why Liver Health Should Be Your Top Priority

Many people take the health of their liver for granted because it doesn't show signs of distress unless the damage is already significant. However, the liver is vital to so many functions of the body that neglecting it can result in serious, long-term health issues.

First, let's think of the liver as a grand filtration system for the body. It is responsible for filtering toxins and waste products from the blood, detoxifying everything from environmental pollutants to the byproducts of alcohol and certain medications. It also regulates cholesterol levels, manufactures proteins, and stores glycogen, which is critical for maintaining steady blood sugar levels. Without a healthy liver, these vital processes cannot function efficiently.

Unfortunately, the liver doesn't come with a warning system. People often continue to feel healthy even when the liver is compromised, and it can take years before the symptoms of liver disease such as fatigue, digestive problems, or skin conditions become noticeable. By then, the liver may already be significantly damaged. This is why liver health should be a top priority—by protecting your liver early, you give yourself the best chance at long-term health and vitality.

Liver dysfunction, including conditions like fatty liver disease, cirrhosis, hepatitis, or even liver cancer, is becoming increasingly common due to poor lifestyle choices, the rise in obesity rates, alcohol consumption, and exposure to toxins. These conditions can lead to liver failure, a life-threatening event that could have been prevented. So, now is the time to start taking proactive steps to protect this crucial organ.

The Role of the Liver in Overall Health

To understand why liver health should be prioritized, we must first appreciate just how essential the liver is in maintaining overall health. This remarkable organ weighs about three pounds in an average adult and performs hundreds of critical functions that allow other systems in the body to function smoothly.

Here are some of the key roles the liver plays in maintaining health:

Table of Contents

1. **Detoxification:** The liver is the body's primary detoxifier. It filters out harmful substances like alcohol, prescription drugs, and environmental toxins from the blood. These toxins could otherwise accumulate and poison the body, leading to illness or organ damage.

2. **Metabolism:** The liver is central to regulating metabolism. It helps process and store nutrients from food, converting them into energy or storing them for later use. It also plays a significant role in controlling blood sugar levels by storing glucose and releasing it when the body needs it.

3. **Bile Production:** The liver produces bile, a substance essential for digesting fats and absorbing fat-soluble vitamins like vitamins A, D, E, and K. Without bile, your body would be unable to process fats, leading to nutritional deficiencies.

4. **Protein Synthesis:** The liver manufactures a number of vital proteins, including albumin (which helps maintain fluid balance in the body) and clotting factors (which are necessary for blood clotting). Without these proteins, your blood wouldn't clot properly, and your body would struggle to maintain its fluid balance.

5. **Storage of Nutrients:** The liver stores important vitamins and minerals like vitamin B12, iron, and copper, making them available to the body when needed. These nutrients are crucial for overall energy production and the proper function of your immune system.

With so many vital functions, it's easy to see why liver health is essential for overall well-being. A compromised liver means the entire system starts to falter, leading to a domino effect that can create a host of health issues throughout the body.

How Liver Dysfunction Impacts the Entire Body

Liver dysfunction is not just confined to one area of the body; it impacts nearly every system. While the liver has an incredible ability to regenerate and heal itself when damage occurs, over time, repeated or continuous damage can lead to irreversible conditions such as cirrhosis or liver failure. Here's how liver dysfunction can affect the body:

1. **Digestive Issues:** Because the liver produces bile, which helps break down fats during digestion, impaired liver function can lead to digestive problems. This may include bloating, diarrhea, constipation, and difficulty digesting fatty foods.

2. **Fatigue and Weakness:** The liver plays a critical role in regulating energy by metabolizing fats, carbohydrates, and proteins. When the liver isn't functioning properly, the body may not be able to extract or store enough energy from food, resulting in chronic fatigue and weakness.

3. **Hormonal Imbalance:** The liver regulates hormones like estrogen, thyroid hormones, and insulin. Dysfunction in the liver can cause hormonal imbalances that lead to a range of symptoms, such as weight gain, mood swings, acne, or irregular periods.

4. **Immune System Dysfunction:** The liver plays a role in modulating the immune system. It produces immune factors and helps clear pathogens from the bloodstream. If the liver isn't working properly, the immune system

becomes less efficient, making the body more susceptible to infections.

5. **Skin Problems:** When the liver can't efficiently remove toxins from the body, these toxins can accumulate and manifest as skin problems. Conditions like acne, rashes, jaundice (yellowing of the skin), and even eczema can all be signs of liver dysfunction.

6. **Mental Fog and Cognitive Decline:** The liver is responsible for processing and clearing out ammonia, a toxic substance produced by the body. If the liver is compromised, ammonia builds up in the bloodstream, which can lead to confusion, memory problems, and other cognitive issues.

7. **Weight Gain and Obesity:** One of the most significant consequences of liver dysfunction is the inability to properly metabolize and store fats. This can result in weight gain, particularly in the abdominal area, and is one of the hallmarks of conditions like fatty liver disease.

Understanding the Signs and Symptoms of Liver Problems

As I mentioned earlier, the liver often doesn't show signs of distress until significant damage has occurred. However, there are several common symptoms that may indicate liver problems. These symptoms can be subtle at first, but they should never be ignored:

1. **Fatigue:** Chronic fatigue and a lack of energy are often the first noticeable symptoms of liver dysfunction. Since the

liver is involved in energy metabolism, a malfunctioning liver can make you feel constantly tired and drained.

2. **Jaundice:** One of the most apparent signs of liver disease is jaundice, which is the yellowing of the skin or eyes. This occurs when the liver cannot process bilirubin, a byproduct of red blood cell breakdown.

3. **Digestive Issues:** Indigestion, bloating, nausea, and loss of appetite can be signs of liver problems. If the liver isn't producing enough bile or is struggling to process food, these digestive disturbances may occur.

4. **Swelling in the Abdomen or Legs:** Liver dysfunction can cause fluid to accumulate in the abdomen (ascites) and legs (edema), making the body appear swollen and puffy.

5. **Dark Urine and Pale Stools:** If the liver is unable to process bile properly, it may lead to changes in urine and stool color. Dark urine and pale stools are common signs of liver issues.

6. **Itchy Skin:** Chronic itching, or pruritus, is often linked to liver disease, particularly when bile flow is obstructed.

7. **Easy Bruising and Bleeding:** Since the liver produces clotting factors, liver dysfunction can lead to easy bruising, excessive bleeding, and prolonged recovery after injury.

If you experience any of these symptoms, it is crucial to consult a healthcare professional to get the proper diagnosis and treatment.

Why You Need to Act Now to Protect Your Liver

Now that we understand how critical liver health is, it's time to address the most important point—why you need to take action now. As mentioned earlier, liver dysfunction often develops silently, and by the time symptoms appear, the damage may be irreversible. Here are a few compelling reasons why you must protect your liver today:

1. **Liver Disease Is on the Rise:** Conditions like fatty liver disease, cirrhosis, and liver cancer are becoming more common due to poor dietary habits, sedentary lifestyles, and environmental toxins. You don't want to be part of these statistics—acting now can prevent the onset of disease.

2. **The Liver Has Limited Warning Signs:** As the liver doesn't exhibit obvious signs of dysfunction until it's too late, early prevention is key. By making small lifestyle changes today—such as improving your diet, reducing alcohol intake, and managing stress—you can safeguard your liver from future damage.

3. **Your Liver Is Vital for Your Quality of Life:** If you're serious about maintaining overall health and vitality, your liver cannot be neglected. You can't afford to wait until liver disease takes hold. Protecting your liver now is the best thing you can do for your future health.

By understanding the importance of the liver, recognizing the symptoms of dysfunction, and making proactive lifestyle changes, you're on your way to a healthier, longer life. Your liver is one of the most vital organs in your body, and it deserves your utmost care and attention.

Chapter 1: The Basics of Liver Health

The liver, one of the most vital organs in the human body, is often underappreciated. Hidden beneath the rib cage, it works tirelessly to support many of the body's most crucial functions. If you are serious about improving your health and longevity, understanding the role of the liver should be your first step. A healthy liver is essential to your well-being and can directly influence your quality of life.

What is the Liver and What Does It Do?

The liver is a large, reddish-brown organ located in the upper right side of the abdomen, beneath the diaphragm. It weighs around 3 pounds and is roughly the size of a football. Despite its relatively small size compared to other organs, the liver performs over 500 essential tasks that are vital for the body's normal functioning. It is the only organ capable of regenerating itself, which is why it is so resilient, even in the face of significant damage.

The liver is often compared to a power station, where several crucial metabolic processes occur. These processes include detoxification, nutrient storage, blood filtration, and enzyme production. It also plays a vital role in regulating vital aspects of bodily functions like digestion and metabolism. In essence, the liver is like a behind-the-scenes manager, ensuring everything runs smoothly, without us even noticing.

Overview of the Liver's Functions

The liver is responsible for a wide array of functions that support overall health. Below are some of the key functions:

1. **Detoxification**

   The liver detoxifies harmful substances in the body by breaking them down and neutralizing toxins, such as alcohol, drugs, and pollutants. It processes these toxins through specialized enzymes, making them safe to be eliminated from the body. This function is vital because our bodies are constantly exposed to environmental toxins, chemicals in food, and waste produced from daily metabolic activities.

2. **Metabolism**

   The liver plays a crucial role in converting the food we eat into energy. It helps in digesting carbohydrates, fats, and proteins and converting them into glucose, which is used by the body for energy. Additionally, the liver regulates the release of glucose from the blood when levels are too high or stores glucose for future energy needs when levels drop.

3. **Storage of Nutrients**

   The liver stores essential vitamins (A, D, B12), minerals (iron, copper), and glucose in the form of glycogen. These nutrients are stored in the liver for later use when the body needs them for energy, or to maintain bodily functions. The liver is also responsible for storing and releasing cholesterol, which is needed for producing hormones and other vital functions.

4. **Protein Synthesis**

   One of the most important roles the liver plays is the production of proteins essential for health. For example, the liver produces blood-clotting proteins, albumin (which helps maintain blood volume), and enzymes that are vital for metabolic processes. Without the liver's ability to create proteins, the body would struggle to perform basic functions like blood clotting, immune defense, and cell repair.

5. **Bile Production**
   Bile, a fluid produced by the liver, is essential for digestion and absorption of fats and fat-soluble vitamins. Once produced in the liver, bile is stored in the gallbladder and then released into the small intestine to aid in digestion. Without bile, the body would struggle to digest fats properly, leading to deficiencies and digestive issues.

Detoxification and Metabolism

The liver is often referred to as the body's detoxification center because it processes and eliminates harmful substances. Detoxification is an intricate process carried out by the liver's various enzymes and biochemical pathways. The liver breaks down toxins like alcohol, drugs, and metabolic waste, neutralizing them to prevent harm to the body.

The liver's detoxification process involves two phases:

- **Phase 1: Activation**
  In this phase, the liver uses enzymes to break down toxic substances into smaller, potentially more reactive molecules. While this process may make toxins less harmful, it can sometimes create new toxic byproducts that need to be dealt with in Phase 2.

- **Phase 2: Conjugation**
  During this phase, the liver neutralizes the byproducts produced in Phase 1 by attaching them to other substances, making them water-soluble. These water-soluble

substances are then excreted through the kidneys or intestines in urine or bile. This is how the body gets rid of harmful chemicals and waste products.

Metabolism, on the other hand, is the process by which your body turns food into energy. The liver plays a critical role in regulating metabolism by converting excess glucose into glycogen, which is stored for future use. When blood sugar levels drop, the liver releases glycogen, converting it back into glucose to maintain energy balance. Similarly, the liver metabolizes fats into fatty acids and lipoproteins, which are essential for hormone production and cell function.

Digestive Role: How the Liver Supports Your Gut Health

While the liver itself doesn't directly participate in digestion, it plays an indispensable role in supporting gut health. Its digestive function is centered around the production and secretion of bile, a substance that is critical for the digestion and absorption of fats.

Bile is produced by liver cells, called hepatocytes, and stored in the gallbladder. When you eat foods containing fats, bile is released into the small intestine to emulsify the fats, breaking them down into smaller droplets that are easier to absorb. Without enough bile, the digestive system cannot effectively break down fats, leading to issues such as malabsorption, nutrient deficiencies, and digestive discomfort.

Additionally, the liver processes nutrients absorbed through the intestines. After you eat, nutrients from food enter the bloodstream through the small intestine. The blood then travels to the liver through the portal vein, where the liver filters and processes these nutrients. For example, after you eat carbohydrates, the liver converts excess glucose into glycogen and stores it. The liver also detoxifies any potentially harmful substances absorbed by the intestines, helping protect the body from toxins that could cause illness.

The Importance of the Liver in Blood Sugar Regulation

Blood sugar regulation is one of the liver's most critical functions. The liver helps maintain stable blood sugar levels, which is essential for overall health. When you eat, the body absorbs glucose from food, raising blood sugar levels. The liver helps regulate these levels by either storing glucose for later use or releasing it into the bloodstream when levels are too low.

When blood sugar levels rise after eating, the liver stores glucose in the form of glycogen, helping lower blood sugar levels back to normal. When blood sugar levels drop, the liver converts stored glycogen back into glucose and releases it into the bloodstream, ensuring that the body always has a steady supply of energy.

The liver is also involved in the conversion of excess glucose into fat when there is an overabundance of sugar in the bloodstream. This stored fat can be used as a long-term energy reserve. However, excessive storage of fat in the liver, as seen in conditions like fatty liver disease, can lead to health problems and disrupt the liver's ability to regulate blood sugar.

In addition to regulating blood glucose levels, the liver also plays a role in managing insulin sensitivity. Insulin is a hormone that helps cells absorb glucose from the bloodstream. The liver helps balance insulin levels by regulating how much glucose is released into the bloodstream. Insulin resistance, often linked to obesity and metabolic syndrome, can occur when the liver becomes overwhelmed and is no longer able to respond properly to insulin signals.

Common Liver Diseases and Their Impact

The liver is one of the most vital organs in our body, performing a variety of essential functions such as detoxification, metabolism, nutrient storage, and blood clotting. However, like all organs, the liver can be susceptible to diseases that affect its ability to perform these functions properly. Liver diseases are common and can range from mild, asymptomatic conditions to severe, life-threatening diseases.

Liver disease can affect individuals of all ages, and the impact of these diseases can be both immediate and long-term. Liver diseases are often categorized based on the cause, such as viral infections, alcohol use, obesity, and autoimmune conditions, among others. Understanding these diseases is crucial because many liver diseases, especially in their early stages, can go unnoticed until they progress into something more serious.

Fatty Liver Disease (NAFLD & NASH)

Non-alcoholic Fatty Liver Disease (NAFLD) and **Non-alcoholic Steatohepatitis (NASH)** are two of the most common liver diseases today. Both are part of a spectrum of conditions associated with the accumulation of fat in liver cells, which is unrelated to alcohol consumption. The cause of fat accumulation in the liver often ties to obesity, poor diet, lack of exercise, and metabolic disorders like diabetes.

NAFLD (Non-Alcoholic Fatty Liver Disease)

NAFLD is the milder form of fatty liver disease. It occurs when excess fat accumulates in the liver, but there is no inflammation or liver damage. In the early stages, most individuals with NAFLD show no symptoms and the condition may go undetected without routine liver function tests.

The risk factors for NAFLD include:

- **Obesity**: Excess body fat, especially around the abdomen, can increase the risk of fat buildup in the liver.
- **Type 2 Diabetes**: Insulin resistance is often associated with NAFLD.
- **High cholesterol and high blood pressure**: These conditions are also risk factors for developing fatty liver disease.
- **Poor diet**: Diets high in refined sugars, unhealthy fats, and processed foods can contribute to the condition.
- **Sedentary lifestyle**: Lack of physical activity contributes to obesity and metabolic disorders.

Though NAFLD does not necessarily cause liver damage on its own, it can progress over time into a more severe form, leading to inflammation and scarring of the liver.

NASH (Non-Alcoholic Steatohepatitis)

NASH is a more severe form of NAFLD. In NASH, the liver not only accumulates fat, but also experiences inflammation and liver cell damage. NASH can lead to scarring of the liver, also known as **fibrosis**. As fibrosis progresses, it can eventually lead to **cirrhosis**, liver failure, and other life-threatening complications.

The progression from NAFLD to NASH is not inevitable, but certain risk factors can increase the likelihood of it happening, including prolonged obesity, uncontrolled diabetes, and other metabolic issues. People with NASH are at greater risk of developing liver cancer, so early detection and intervention are critical.

Cirrhosis

Cirrhosis is the term for the late-stage scarring (fibrosis) of the liver caused by continuous injury and long-term liver disease. It is often a result of chronic liver conditions such as fatty liver disease, hepatitis, and excessive alcohol use.

In cirrhosis, healthy liver tissue is replaced by scar tissue, which obstructs the normal flow of blood through the liver and impairs its ability to function. The liver's ability to perform essential functions, like detoxifying chemicals, producing important proteins, and regulating blood clotting, becomes significantly diminished.

Causes of Cirrhosis

- **Chronic alcohol use**: Alcohol consumption is one of the leading causes of cirrhosis. Over time, excessive drinking leads to liver inflammation, fat accumulation, and ultimately, cirrhosis.
- **Viral hepatitis**: Chronic infections caused by the hepatitis viruses (B, C) can cause ongoing liver damage and cirrhosis.
- **Fatty liver disease**: Both NAFLD and NASH can contribute to the development of cirrhosis when left untreated.

- **Medications and toxins**: Long-term use of certain medications or exposure to toxic substances can also damage the liver.
- **Autoimmune liver diseases**: Conditions such as autoimmune hepatitis can lead to cirrhosis.

Symptoms and Impact of Cirrhosis

In the early stages, cirrhosis may have no symptoms. As the disease progresses, symptoms can include:

- **Fatigue**
- **Jaundice (yellowing of the skin and eyes)**
- **Abdominal pain**
- **Swelling in the abdomen or legs**
- **Confusion or difficulty thinking clearly (hepatic encephalopathy)**

Cirrhosis can lead to serious complications, including liver failure, bleeding disorders, and liver cancer. Early diagnosis and management of cirrhosis can slow the progression of the disease, but the condition is irreversible once scarring occurs.

Hepatitis (A, B, C)

Hepatitis refers to inflammation of the liver, typically caused by viral infections. There are several types of viral hepatitis, with **Hepatitis A**, **Hepatitis B**, and **Hepatitis C** being the most common.

Hepatitis A

Hepatitis A is a viral infection caused by the Hepatitis A virus (HAV), which is typically transmitted through contaminated food or water, or close personal contact with an infected person. Hepatitis A causes acute liver inflammation but usually does not lead to chronic liver disease.

- **Symptoms**: Jaundice, fatigue, nausea, abdominal pain, and dark-colored urine.
- **Prevention**: The Hepatitis A vaccine is widely available and is the most effective prevention method.
- **Prognosis**: Most people with Hepatitis A recover fully within a few months, though in rare cases, the infection can cause liver failure.

Hepatitis B

Hepatitis B is caused by the Hepatitis B virus (HBV) and is transmitted through blood, semen, or other bodily fluids. It can be passed through unprotected sex, sharing needles, or from mother to baby during birth.

- **Acute vs Chronic**: Hepatitis B can be either acute (short-term) or chronic (long-term). Chronic Hepatitis B can lead to cirrhosis and liver cancer if left untreated.
- **Symptoms**: Jaundice, fatigue, joint pain, abdominal pain, and dark urine. However, many people with Hepatitis B show no symptoms.
- **Prevention**: The Hepatitis B vaccine is highly effective in preventing the infection.
- **Treatment**: Antiviral medications can help control the infection, but there is no cure for chronic Hepatitis B.

Hepatitis C

Hepatitis C is caused by the Hepatitis C virus (HCV) and is primarily transmitted through blood-to-blood contact, such as sharing needles or receiving blood transfusions before 1992.

- **Chronic Infection**: Hepatitis C is often chronic and can lead to liver cirrhosis and liver cancer if left untreated.
- **Symptoms**: Similar to Hepatitis B, many people with Hepatitis C show no symptoms until liver damage becomes significant.
- **Treatment**: There are highly effective antiviral treatments available that can cure most cases of Hepatitis C.
- **Prevention**: There is no vaccine for Hepatitis C, but the spread of the virus can be prevented by avoiding sharing needles and practicing safe sex.

Liver Cancer

Liver cancer is one of the deadliest cancers worldwide, and its incidence has been rising in recent years. The most common form of liver cancer is **hepatocellular carcinoma (HCC)**, which typically develops in individuals with chronic liver diseases such as cirrhosis or Hepatitis B or C infection.

Risk Factors

- **Chronic liver disease**: Conditions such as cirrhosis, hepatitis, and fatty liver disease significantly increase the risk of liver cancer.
- **Alcohol consumption**: Chronic heavy drinking can increase the risk of liver cancer, particularly in individuals with cirrhosis.
- **Obesity and Diabetes**: Metabolic conditions such as obesity and type 2 diabetes can increase the risk of liver cancer.
- **Exposure to aflatoxins**: These toxins, produced by certain molds, can increase the risk of liver cancer, particularly in parts of the world where food is not stored properly.

Symptoms

- **Pain in the upper abdomen**
- **Unexplained weight loss**
- **Jaundice**
- **Fatigue**
- **Nausea or vomiting**

Liver cancer is often diagnosed at a later stage, making it difficult to treat. However, treatments such as surgery, liver transplantation, and chemotherapy can improve survival rates.

Autoimmune Liver Diseases

Autoimmune liver diseases occur when the body's immune system mistakenly attacks its own liver cells, causing inflammation and damage. The most common autoimmune liver diseases are **autoimmune hepatitis**, **primary biliary cirrhosis (PBC)**, and **primary sclerosing cholangitis (PSC)**.

Autoimmune Hepatitis

In autoimmune hepatitis, the immune system targets and attacks the liver cells, causing inflammation. This condition can be mild or severe and may lead to cirrhosis if left untreated.

- **Symptoms**: Fatigue, jaundice, abdominal pain, joint pain, and an enlarged liver.
- **Treatment**: Immunosuppressive medications, such as corticosteroids, are commonly used to control the condition and prevent further liver damage.

Primary Biliary Cirrhosis (PBC)

PBC is a chronic autoimmune condition where the immune system attacks the bile ducts in the liver. Over time, this causes liver damage and cirrhosis.

- **Symptoms**: Fatigue, itchy skin, jaundice, and dry eyes or mouth.
- **Treatment**: Ursodeoxycholic acid is the standard treatment to slow disease progression.

Primary Sclerosing Cholangitis (PSC)

PSC is a rare autoimmune condition that causes inflammation and scarring of the bile ducts. This can lead to cirrhosis and liver failure.

- **Symptoms**: Similar to PBC, including fatigue, jaundice, and itching.
- **Treatment**: There is no cure for PSC, but medications and liver transplantation may help manage symptoms.

Chapter 2: How Modern Life Damages the Liver

The liver is a vital organ that plays an integral role in keeping the body healthy. It's responsible for filtering toxins, producing bile to help digest fat, storing vitamins and minerals, and much more. However, in modern life, the liver is subjected to numerous factors that can damage its delicate functions. These factors include poor diet, excessive consumption of alcohol, environmental toxins, and the overuse of medications. In this chapter, we'll explore how modern lifestyle habits are putting our liver at risk.

Diet and Its Effects on Liver Health

In today's fast-paced world, many people are accustomed to eating on the go, opting for quick meals that are not necessarily the healthiest options. Unfortunately, this convenience often comes at a high cost to liver health. The foods we eat have a direct impact on how well our liver functions. The liver is responsible for breaking down and processing everything we consume, which means it's affected by our dietary choices, whether positive or negative.

Unhealthy Fats and Their Impact

One of the biggest culprits when it comes to liver health is the consumption of unhealthy fats. These fats, found in processed foods like fast food, pastries, and fried foods, can lead to the buildup of fat within the liver. Over time, this fat accumulation can develop into fatty liver disease, a condition that can severely impact liver function. Non-alcoholic fatty liver disease (NAFLD) is one of the most common liver conditions today, largely due to diets high in unhealthy fats.

The liver can handle small amounts of fat, but an overload can lead to inflammation, which causes further damage. If left unchecked, fatty liver can progress to cirrhosis, a condition where the liver becomes scarred and is no longer able to perform its necessary functions.

The Role of Sugar and Carbohydrates

Excessive sugar and refined carbohydrates, such as white bread, pasta, and sugary drinks, can have an equally harmful effect on liver health. When consumed in large quantities, sugar is converted into fat in the liver. This contributes to the same fat accumulation that can lead to fatty liver disease. In fact, high sugar intake has been linked to the development of both non-alcoholic fatty liver disease (NAFLD) and insulin resistance.

Refined carbohydrates have a similar effect. They spike blood sugar levels, which can lead to the release of insulin. Chronic high levels of insulin can promote fat storage in the liver, further exacerbating the risk of liver disease.

Processed Foods, Sugars, and Their Impact

In the modern diet, processed foods have become staples. Foods such as packaged snacks, ready-to-eat meals, and sugary beverages often contain preservatives, artificial sweeteners, and high amounts of unhealthy fats and sugar. These ingredients can have a profound impact on liver health.

Artificial Additives and Toxins

Many processed foods are packed with artificial additives like colorings, preservatives, and flavor enhancers. These chemicals are often absorbed into the body, putting additional stress on the liver.

The liver works hard to detoxify these substances, but when the body is constantly exposed to a high level of toxins from processed foods, it can become overwhelmed.

Artificial sweeteners, such as aspartame and sucralose, are commonly found in diet sodas and sugar-free snacks. While these sweeteners are marketed as healthy alternatives to sugar, research has shown that they can disrupt liver metabolism. Some studies have linked them to liver damage and the development of fatty liver disease.

High Fructose Corn Syrup (HFCS)

Another problematic ingredient in many processed foods is high fructose corn syrup (HFCS). Found in many sodas, snacks, and baked goods, HFCS is a highly processed form of sugar that is particularly harmful to the liver. Research has shown that the liver metabolizes fructose differently than glucose, causing it to store more fat. This fat accumulation can lead to the development of fatty liver disease and increase the risk of metabolic disorders such as obesity and diabetes.

The liver is designed to process small amounts of sugar, but excessive intake of fructose can overload the organ, resulting in inflammation and oxidative stress. This damages liver cells and contributes to long-term liver problems.

Alcohol Consumption and Liver Disease

Alcohol is one of the leading causes of liver disease around the world. The liver is responsible for metabolizing alcohol, but excessive and chronic consumption can overwhelm its ability to detoxify. Over time, this can lead to liver inflammation, cirrhosis, and other serious health complications.

How Alcohol Affects the Liver

When you drink alcohol, the liver breaks it down into acetaldehyde, a toxic substance that can cause inflammation in the liver cells. Acetaldehyde is then further broken down into acetic acid, which is eventually processed and eliminated from the body. However, if alcohol is consumed in large quantities over time, the liver becomes unable to detoxify efficiently. The excess alcohol can lead to fatty liver disease, alcoholic hepatitis, and eventually cirrhosis.

The Dangers of Heavy Drinking

Heavy drinking places a significant strain on the liver. Chronic alcohol abuse can lead to alcoholic fatty liver disease (AFLD), which is characterized by fat accumulation in liver cells. Over time, this can progress to alcoholic hepatitis, a condition where the liver becomes inflamed. If left untreated, alcoholic hepatitis can result in cirrhosis, a potentially life-threatening condition where liver cells become scarred and unable to regenerate.

It's important to note that alcohol-related liver disease is not limited to those who drink excessively. Even moderate drinking can have an impact on liver health over time, especially when combined with poor diet and other lifestyle factors.

The Dangers of Excessive Medications

While medications are often necessary for treating health conditions, excessive or improper use of certain medications can damage the liver. The liver plays a crucial role in metabolizing drugs, and when the body is overloaded with medications, it can lead to liver toxicity.

Over-the-Counter Painkillers

Common over-the-counter (OTC) painkillers like acetaminophen (Tylenol) are among the most widely used medications. However, taking high doses of acetaminophen can overwhelm the liver's detoxification system and cause liver damage. This is particularly true if the drug is taken in conjunction with alcohol or other medications that also put stress on the liver. Acute liver failure from acetaminophen overdose is a leading cause of liver transplants in the United States.

Prescription Medications

Prescription medications, especially those taken over long periods, can also have a harmful effect on liver health. Statins, which are commonly prescribed to lower cholesterol, have been shown to cause liver damage in some individuals. Additionally, antibiotics, anti-inflammatory drugs, and other prescription medications can increase the risk of liver injury.

Some people are genetically predisposed to having a heightened sensitivity to certain medications. In these cases, even standard doses can cause severe liver damage. It's essential for individuals to follow their healthcare provider's guidance when taking medications and to monitor liver function regularly if prescribed long-term treatment.

Herbal Supplements and Interactions

Although herbal supplements are often marketed as natural remedies, they can also pose a risk to liver health. Some herbs, such as kava, comfrey, and chaparral, have been linked to liver toxicity. Additionally, herbal supplements can interact with prescription medications, amplifying their effects and leading to liver damage. It's important to inform your healthcare provider about any supplements you're taking to avoid harmful interactions.

Environmental Toxins and Liver Stress

As an experienced healthcare professional, I've seen time and again how environmental toxins wreak havoc on our bodies, and most notably, on the liver. The liver is our primary detoxification organ; its job is to filter harmful substances from the blood, detoxify chemicals, and break down metabolic waste. However, the sheer volume and variety of environmental toxins that we encounter on a daily basis place incredible strain on this organ, leaving it vulnerable to diseases and conditions.

Environmental toxins come from a wide range of sources, from industrial waste to chemicals in the food and water supply. Let's examine the key sources of these toxins, how they affect liver health, and what can be done to reduce their impact.

The Scope of Environmental Toxins

Environmental toxins can be divided into several categories, each contributing to liver stress in different ways.

1. **Air Pollution**
    The air we breathe is filled with pollutants that can cause harm to the liver. From vehicle emissions to industrial exhaust, fine particulate matter (PM2.5) and toxic gases like carbon monoxide and nitrogen dioxide are common in polluted areas. These pollutants not only irritate the respiratory system but also make their way into the bloodstream, eventually reaching the liver, where they are processed. Continuous exposure to these harmful particles can lead to chronic inflammation in the liver, making it more difficult for the organ to detoxify effectively.

2. **Pesticides and Herbicides**

Pesticides and herbicides used in agriculture are another significant source of toxins that affect liver health. While these chemicals are designed to kill pests and weeds, they also have a toxic effect on humans. Many pesticides contain organophosphates and other chemicals that are highly toxic to the liver. These substances accumulate over time in the body, placing added pressure on the liver's detoxification systems and increasing the risk of liver disease.

3. **Industrial Chemicals and Waste**

Chemicals like solvents, plastics, and volatile organic compounds (VOCs) found in household products can accumulate in the body and cause liver strain. Industrial waste, including by-products from manufacturing processes, can leak into the air, water, and soil, spreading toxic substances into our communities. Long-term exposure to these pollutants has been linked to liver cirrhosis, hepatitis, and even liver cancer.

4. **Pharmaceutical Pollution**

In recent years, pharmaceutical residues have been detected in drinking water sources and even in the air we breathe. These pharmaceutical contaminants can come from improperly discarded medications or from drugs that pass through the human body and are excreted in urine. The liver is responsible for metabolizing many drugs, but a build-up of pharmaceutical toxins in the body can overwhelm the liver's ability to detoxify, leading to liver stress and increased vulnerability to disease.

How Environmental Toxins Harm the Liver

The liver functions as a filtration system, processing toxins and waste products from the bloodstream. However, when the liver is bombarded by toxins from the environment, its detoxification capacity becomes compromised. The overload of chemicals, heavy metals, and pollutants triggers an inflammatory response in the liver. This inflammation leads to liver cell damage, a decrease in liver function, and, over time, the development of liver diseases such as fatty liver disease and cirrhosis.

1. **Inflammation and Oxidative Stress**

    Many environmental toxins, especially air pollutants and chemicals, cause oxidative stress in liver cells. This happens when harmful free radicals are produced faster than the liver can neutralize them. These free radicals damage liver cells and tissues, making them more susceptible to inflammation. Chronic inflammation is one of the leading causes of liver damage and disease.

2. **Fatty Liver Disease**

    Exposure to environmental toxins can also contribute to the development of fatty liver disease. This occurs when harmful substances cause the liver to store excess fat, leading to liver dysfunction. Fatty liver disease is often asymptomatic in the early stages, but over time, it can progress to more serious conditions such as cirrhosis or liver failure.

3. **Liver Cancer**

    Long-term exposure to environmental carcinogens, such as pesticides, industrial chemicals, and pharmaceutical pollutants, increases the risk of liver cancer. These substances can cause mutations in liver cells, leading to the development of cancerous growths.

Reducing Liver Stress from Environmental Toxins

While it's impossible to completely avoid exposure to environmental toxins, there are steps that can be taken to reduce their impact on liver health:

- **Limit Exposure**: Reduce exposure to air pollution by staying indoors on high pollution days. Opt for organic foods to avoid pesticides, and make efforts to reduce household chemical use by choosing natural cleaning products.
- **Detoxification**: Regular detoxification strategies such as consuming liver-supporting foods (e.g., garlic, leafy greens, and turmeric) and staying hydrated can help support the liver's detoxification processes.
- **Supportive Supplements**: Milk thistle and other liver-supportive supplements can help repair liver cells and reduce the oxidative stress caused by environmental toxins.
- **Healthy Lifestyle Choices**: Exercise regularly to help the body eliminate toxins through sweat and improve overall liver health. Eating a balanced diet rich in antioxidants and anti-inflammatory foods can also help protect the liver.

By understanding the connection between environmental toxins and liver stress, you can take proactive steps to minimize your exposure and support liver health.

Household Chemicals and Pollution

Many of us believe that our homes are safe havens, free from the harmful pollutants that might exist outside. However, the truth is that household chemicals and pollution are often far more harmful than we realize, particularly when it comes to our liver health. Our homes are filled with chemicals in cleaning products, paints, personal care items, and even furniture. Over time, exposure to these chemicals can add significant stress to the liver, hindering its ability to perform its crucial detoxifying functions.

Common Household Chemicals

1. **Cleaning Products**

   Household cleaning products, such as bleach, ammonia, and various disinfectants, often contain toxic chemicals that are absorbed through the skin or inhaled. These substances can cause irritation and inflammation in the liver, overwhelming its detoxification capacity. Many cleaning products also contain volatile organic compounds (VOCs), which can lead to liver cell damage when they accumulate in the body.

2. **Air Fresheners and Candles**

   Air fresheners, including sprays, plug-ins, and scented candles, often contain chemicals like phthalates, formaldehyde, and synthetic fragrances that have been linked to liver damage. Prolonged exposure to these substances can contribute to liver inflammation and oxidative stress, weakening the liver's ability to process toxins.

3. **Cosmetics and Personal Care Products**

   Many cosmetics and personal care products, such as shampoos, lotions, and makeup, contain harmful chemicals like parabens, sulfates, and phthalates. These substances can be absorbed into the bloodstream through the skin, making their way to the liver, where they are metabolized. Over time, the accumulation of these chemicals can increase liver stress and hinder its detoxification processes.

4. **Pesticides and Herbicides**
   While these chemicals are used outside to control pests and weeds, they can also find their way into the home through food or indoor plants. Pesticides like organophosphates have been shown to disrupt liver function, leading to a host of health problems over time.

How Household Chemicals Affect the Liver

The liver is tasked with filtering and breaking down many of the chemicals we come into contact with, but when it's overwhelmed by the sheer volume of pollutants from household products, it can't keep up. The result is an increase in liver inflammation, oxidative stress, and an overall decline in liver function.

1. **Toxin Build-Up**
   Chemicals found in household products often accumulate in the liver. Over time, this build-up can lead to fatty liver disease, liver fibrosis, or even cirrhosis if left unchecked.

2. **Hormonal Disruption**
   Many household chemicals, particularly those in personal care products, act as endocrine disruptors. These disruptors interfere with the body's hormonal balance, which can affect liver function. The liver plays a crucial role in hormone regulation, and exposure to chemicals that interfere with this process can lead to liver dysfunction.

3. **Inflammation and Immune Response**
   The liver is integral to the immune system, filtering out pathogens and chemicals that could harm the body. Chronic exposure to household toxins increases liver inflammation, which can impair the immune system's ability to function

effectively.

How to Protect Your Liver from Household Chemicals

- **Go Natural**: Choose natural cleaning products free from harmful chemicals. You can make your own cleaning solutions with simple ingredients like vinegar, baking soda, and lemon.
- **Use Non-Toxic Cosmetics**: Opt for organic and non-toxic personal care products that are free from parabens, sulfates, and synthetic fragrances.
- **Ventilate Your Home**: Ensure proper ventilation to reduce the concentration of harmful fumes in your home. Regularly open windows and use air purifiers to improve indoor air quality.
- **Wash Produce Thoroughly**: Always wash fruits and vegetables thoroughly to remove any pesticide residue before eating them.

By making small changes to the chemicals we use in our homes, we can significantly reduce the burden on our liver and improve overall health.

Heavy Metals and Other Harmful Substances

Heavy metals such as mercury, lead, arsenic, and cadmium are among the most harmful substances to the liver. These metals accumulate in the body over time, with the liver acting as the primary organ responsible for filtering and excreting these toxins. When the liver is overburdened with heavy metals, its ability to detoxify the body is compromised, leading to an increased risk of liver disease.

Sources of Heavy Metals

1. **Food and Water**
   Heavy metals can enter our bodies through the food we eat and the water we drink. Contaminated water sources or fish that have been exposed to polluted oceans can be a major source of heavy metals. In particular, fish like tuna, swordfish, and salmon can contain high levels of mercury.

2. **Occupational Exposure**
   Certain jobs, especially in industries like mining, construction, and manufacturing, expose workers to high levels of heavy metals. Inhaling fumes or dust containing metals like lead or arsenic can be particularly harmful to the liver.

3. **Environmental Pollution**
   Heavy metals are often released into the environment through industrial activities and waste disposal. These metals can contaminate soil and water, eventually making their way into the food chain.

4. **Cosmetics and Household Items**
   Some cosmetics, particularly those containing pigments, as well as household items like batteries, may contain heavy metals like cadmium and lead. Prolonged exposure to these metals can lead to liver damage and other health problems.

How Heavy Metals Harm the Liver

Heavy metals are toxic to liver cells, causing a range of issues from cellular damage to full-blown liver diseases. The liver's detoxification processes can be overwhelmed by the accumulation of these metals, leading to inflammation, fibrosis, and even cancer in some cases.

1. **Oxidative Stress and Inflammation**
   Heavy metals generate free radicals, which cause oxidative stress and inflammation in the liver. Over time, this damages liver cells, impairing their ability to function properly.

2. **Disruption of Liver Enzymes**
   Heavy metals interfere with the enzymes responsible for detoxification in the liver. When these enzymes are compromised, the liver's ability to break down and eliminate toxins is severely reduced.

3. **Fatty Liver Disease and Cirrhosis**
   Long-term exposure to heavy metals increases the risk of developing fatty liver disease, cirrhosis, and even liver cancer. These conditions often go undiagnosed until they reach advanced stages, making early prevention critical.

Reducing Exposure to Heavy Metals

- **Eat Safe Fish**: Choose fish with lower mercury content, such as salmon and sardines, and avoid larger fish like shark and swordfish.
- **Install Water Filtration Systems**: Use a water filter that removes heavy metals from your drinking water to reduce exposure.

- **Avoid Toxic Products**: Be cautious of cosmetics, jewelry, and household items that may contain heavy metals like lead or cadmium.
- **Chelation Therapy**: In some cases, chelation therapy may be used to help remove heavy metals from the body under the supervision of a healthcare provider.

By being aware of the sources of heavy metals and taking preventive measures, we can significantly reduce their harmful effects on the liver and overall health.

Lifestyle Habits That Put Your Liver at Risk

The liver, one of the most vital organs in your body, plays a key role in detoxification, digestion, and energy regulation. However, in today's fast-paced world, many of our lifestyle habits unknowingly place undue stress on our liver. The liver has a remarkable ability to regenerate, but continuous abuse can overwhelm it, leading to chronic conditions such as fatty liver disease, cirrhosis, and even liver cancer.

Some of the most common habits that harm liver health stem from poor diet, sedentary behavior, and excessive substance use. These habits not only affect the liver's natural detoxification process but also reduce its ability to regenerate and function at its best. Let's take a closer look at these harmful lifestyle choices.

1. Excessive Alcohol Consumption

One of the most well-known culprits in liver damage is alcohol. While moderate drinking may not necessarily harm the liver, excessive alcohol consumption leads to liver inflammation, fatty liver, hepatitis, and cirrhosis. Over time, alcohol can overwhelm the liver's ability to metabolize and detoxify it, causing liver cells to die and replace themselves with scar tissue, a condition known as cirrhosis.

Alcoholic beverages, especially when consumed in large quantities, not only burden the liver with the task of detoxifying the alcohol but also trigger inflammation, causing further damage. Many individuals don't realize that even moderate drinking over a prolonged period can cause subtle but significant damage to liver function.

2. Poor Diet and Nutritional Deficiencies

Diet is one of the most significant contributors to liver health. A high-fat diet, particularly one rich in processed foods and sugars, places a great deal of strain on the liver. Foods rich in unhealthy fats and sugar, such as fast food, sugary beverages, and processed snacks, contribute to fatty liver disease (non-alcoholic fatty liver disease or NAFLD), a growing problem worldwide.

A poor diet devoid of essential nutrients such as vitamins, minerals, and antioxidants further impairs liver function. The liver is responsible for processing everything we consume, and a diet lacking in fiber, antioxidants, and healthy fats makes it harder for the liver to detoxify and regenerate. The overconsumption of sugars and unhealthy fats can also cause insulin resistance, leading to fatty deposits in the liver.

3. Overuse of Medications

While medications can save lives, their overuse can harm the liver. Certain prescription and over-the-counter medications are known to place stress on the liver, especially when taken in excess or for prolonged periods. Pain relievers like acetaminophen (Tylenol), statins for cholesterol, and certain antibiotics can lead to liver damage if not carefully monitored.

The liver metabolizes most drugs and clears toxins from the body. When this process is overtaxed by excessive medication use, the liver's ability to detoxify and regenerate diminishes. It's essential for individuals to consult with their healthcare provider before taking long-term medications and to always follow the prescribed dosage to minimize liver stress.

4. Tobacco Use

Smoking is another dangerous habit that harms the liver. Although tobacco is often associated with lung disease and cancer, it can also have detrimental effects on the liver. The chemicals in cigarette smoke can cause inflammation and oxidative stress, leading to liver damage over time. Smoking increases the likelihood of liver disease, particularly when combined with alcohol or other risk factors like obesity.

Tobacco accelerates the development of liver fibrosis, the scarring of liver tissue. Research also shows that smoking can interact with other factors like hepatitis C to worsen liver damage.

5. Lack of Physical Activity

Sedentary lifestyles contribute to numerous health problems, and the liver is no exception. Lack of physical activity leads to obesity, which is one of the leading causes of fatty liver disease. Without regular exercise, your body is more likely to accumulate visceral fat around the liver, leading to inflammation and liver dysfunction.

Physical activity helps improve blood flow to the liver, reduces insulin resistance, and encourages the breakdown of stored fat.

Regular exercise, especially aerobic activities like walking, jogging, and swimming, is essential for maintaining a healthy liver.

Sedentary Lifestyle and Fatty Liver

Sedentary behavior is a modern-day epidemic. With the rise of desk jobs, sedentary hobbies, and extended screen time, more people are spending the majority of their days sitting rather than moving. This lack of physical activity has dire consequences on our overall health, especially the liver.

1. The Connection Between Sedentary Behavior and Liver Fat Accumulation

The liver is responsible for processing fats, but when the body becomes inactive, the metabolism slows down. Fatty acids that should be processed and utilized by the body begin to accumulate in the liver, eventually leading to a condition known as **non-alcoholic fatty liver disease (NAFLD)**. NAFLD occurs when fat builds up in liver cells in the absence of alcohol abuse.

Fat accumulation in the liver leads to inflammation, insulin resistance, and oxidative stress. This process can eventually progress to more severe liver conditions, such as cirrhosis or liver cancer. Studies show that individuals with sedentary lifestyles are more likely to develop NAFLD because their bodies cannot metabolize fat efficiently without regular movement.

2. How Inactivity Affects Insulin Resistance

When a person is inactive, their muscles are less sensitive to insulin. As a result, the body produces more insulin to maintain normal blood sugar levels. Elevated insulin levels can promote fat storage in the liver, leading to insulin resistance and an increased risk of fatty liver disease.

Sedentary behavior also contributes to the metabolic syndrome—a cluster of conditions including high blood sugar, high blood pressure, and abnormal cholesterol levels, all of which increase the risk of developing fatty liver disease.

3. Reducing the Risk: Movement is Key

To combat the risks of a sedentary lifestyle, it's crucial to incorporate regular physical activity into your routine. Aerobic exercises like walking, jogging, cycling, and swimming can significantly improve liver health by reducing fat accumulation and increasing insulin sensitivity.

Experts recommend at least 30 minutes of moderate-intensity exercise most days of the week to support liver health. Incorporating movement into your daily routine, even in small doses, can be transformative for both liver function and overall health.

Stress and Its Connection to Liver Health

Stress is an inevitable part of life, but chronic stress is particularly harmful to your liver. The liver is intimately connected to the body's stress response, and prolonged stress can exacerbate liver damage in various ways. Let's explore how stress affects the liver and what can be done to mitigate these effects.

1. The Body's Stress Response and the Liver

When you experience stress, your body activates the **fight-or-flight** response, triggering the release of hormones like cortisol and adrenaline. These hormones are designed to help you respond to immediate danger, but when stress becomes chronic, these hormones remain elevated in the bloodstream, placing excessive strain on the liver.

Cortisol, in particular, has a direct impact on the liver's function. It encourages the liver to produce more glucose to fuel the body's stress response. While this is helpful in an acute situation, chronic cortisol production can lead to increased blood sugar levels and insulin resistance, both of which are risk factors for fatty liver disease.

2. The Impact of Stress on Digestion and Detoxification

Stress also impairs digestion and detoxification. During stressful times, blood flow is diverted from the digestive system to the muscles and brain, leaving the liver and intestines with less blood flow. This reduces the liver's ability to filter out toxins and metabolize nutrients, leading to a build-up of harmful substances in the body.

Stress-induced inflammation can further damage liver cells, leading to long-term liver dysfunction. Prolonged emotional or psychological stress can trigger or worsen conditions such as hepatitis, cirrhosis, and other chronic liver diseases.

3. Managing Stress for Liver Health

To protect your liver from the damaging effects of stress, it's essential to incorporate stress management techniques into your daily life. Practices such as meditation, yoga, deep breathing exercises, and mindfulness can help reduce cortisol levels and improve liver health. Regular physical activity is also a powerful way to manage stress, as exercise helps regulate hormone levels and reduce inflammation.

Sleep and mental relaxation are key components of stress management. Make time for self-care activities, and try to identify the sources of chronic stress in your life to reduce its impact.

Sleep and Recovery: Their Role in Liver Function

Sleep is vital for overall health, but its importance in liver function is often overlooked. The liver, like all organs, requires rest and recovery to perform its many functions effectively. Let's delve into how sleep affects liver health and why adequate rest is essential for maintaining a healthy liver.

1. The Liver's Repair Process During Sleep

During sleep, the body enters a state of repair and recovery. This includes cellular regeneration in organs like the liver, which is constantly detoxifying and metabolizing nutrients. The liver uses the hours of rest to repair damaged cells, regenerate healthy liver tissue, and eliminate toxins that accumulated throughout the day.

Lack of sleep or poor-quality sleep disrupts this restorative process, making it harder for the liver to function properly. Chronic sleep deprivation can contribute to the accumulation of toxins in the liver, leading to inflammation, insulin resistance, and other liver-related issues.

2. Sleep and Hormone Regulation

Sleep plays a crucial role in regulating hormones that impact liver function. Growth hormone, which is released during deep sleep, aids in tissue repair and liver regeneration. Sleep also helps balance insulin and cortisol levels, both of which affect liver health.

Disrupted sleep patterns, on the other hand, can lead to hormonal imbalances, increasing the risk of liver diseases such as fatty liver disease and cirrhosis. Irregular sleep patterns, such as those caused by shift work or sleep disorders like insomnia, have been linked to a higher risk of liver damage.

3. Improving Sleep Quality for Better Liver Health

To support liver health, it's essential to prioritize sleep. Aim for 7-9 hours of quality sleep each night, and establish a consistent sleep routine. Create a sleep-friendly environment by minimizing distractions and ensuring the room is dark and cool. Reducing caffeine intake, especially later in the day, can also help improve sleep quality.

By taking care of your liver with proper rest, you support its vital functions, allowing it to detoxify the body, regulate metabolism, and maintain overall health.

Chapter 3: Signs and Symptoms of a Compromised Liver

The liver, often referred to as the body's "detox center," plays a critical role in maintaining overall health. It is involved in digesting food, storing energy, filtering out toxins, and producing essential proteins and enzymes. As one of the most vital organs in the body, it has an extraordinary ability to regenerate itself when damaged. However, when the liver becomes compromised, its ability to perform these functions declines, which can lead to a variety of symptoms.

Understanding the early signs and symptoms of liver damage is essential for timely intervention and proper medical treatment. Let's look at the **physical symptoms** you should watch for, specifically focusing on fatigue, skin issues, digestive problems, jaundice, abdominal pain, and bloating.

Physical Symptoms to Watch For

A compromised liver often presents with physical symptoms that indicate its functionality is under duress. These physical signs may develop gradually, which makes them difficult to spot at first. However, once you become familiar with what to look for, you can take preventive action and consult your healthcare provider.

1. **Fatigue and Weakness**: One of the earliest and most common signs of liver dysfunction is persistent fatigue. The liver is responsible for filtering toxins from the blood, metabolizing nutrients, and producing energy. When the liver is not functioning properly, toxins can accumulate in the body, leading to feelings of exhaustion, weakness, and

reduced stamina.

2. **Skin Issues**: The liver plays an important role in detoxification, so when it becomes compromised, the body may begin to exhibit a variety of skin issues. These issues can range from simple rashes and acne to more serious conditions like eczema or psoriasis. Liver dysfunction can cause the skin to become dry, itchy, or discolored. A compromised liver may also result in the buildup of waste products, such as bilirubin, which can manifest as changes in the skin's appearance.

3. **Digestive Problems**: A poorly functioning liver can interfere with digestion, leading to various gastrointestinal problems. These can include indigestion, nausea, and bloating. The liver produces bile, which helps break down fats during digestion. When bile production is inadequate, it can result in fat malabsorption, causing discomfort after meals. Diarrhea or constipation may also become more frequent as the liver struggles to maintain its usual digestive duties.

4. **Jaundice: Yellowing of Skin and Eyes**: Jaundice is one of the hallmark signs of liver dysfunction. It occurs when there is an excess of bilirubin in the bloodstream. Bilirubin is a byproduct of the breakdown of red blood cells, and the liver typically processes it for excretion. When the liver is not functioning properly, bilirubin builds up and causes the skin and the whites of the eyes to take on a yellowish tint. This yellowing, called jaundice, is a clear indicator that the liver is in distress.

5. **Abdominal Pain and Bloating**: When the liver becomes enlarged or inflamed, it can cause pain in the upper right

side of the abdomen. This pain is often described as dull, aching, or sharp. Additionally, the liver's inability to process waste and nutrients efficiently can result in bloating, which is a feeling of fullness or discomfort after eating, often accompanied by excessive gas. Abdominal bloating can also be a symptom of liver-related issues, especially if it is persistent or worsens over time.

Now that we've outlined the **physical symptoms** you should be aware of, let's dive deeper into each one, starting with **fatigue, skin issues, and digestive problems**, and then moving on to more serious signs such as jaundice, abdominal pain, and bloating.

Fatigue, Skin Issues, and Digestive Problems

Fatigue

Fatigue is one of the most noticeable symptoms of a liver in trouble. The liver performs several key functions that are essential for maintaining energy levels. It metabolizes food into usable nutrients, filters toxins from the blood, and stores vitamins and minerals that support bodily functions. When the liver becomes overwhelmed by toxins or damaged by diseases like fatty liver disease, cirrhosis, or hepatitis, it is unable to perform these tasks effectively.

As a result, people with liver dysfunction often experience chronic tiredness. This fatigue doesn't necessarily go away with rest and may be accompanied by feelings of weakness. If you notice a drastic drop in your energy levels, especially if it's accompanied by other signs of liver problems, it is important to seek medical attention.

Skin Issues

The liver plays an important role in detoxification. When the liver isn't functioning properly, the body's toxin levels can rise, which in turn may affect the skin. Some common skin conditions that may occur due to liver issues include:

- **Itchy Skin**: This condition, known as pruritus, occurs when the liver fails to filter bile salts properly. These salts can accumulate under the skin, leading to itching.
- **Rashes**: Individuals with liver disease may develop rashes or red, inflamed areas of skin. These rashes are often the result of toxin buildup or improper bile flow.
- **Discoloration**: The liver's inability to process certain waste products can lead to changes in skin color. Skin may appear blotchy, or you might notice an overall dull complexion. These changes are typically due to the accumulation of bilirubin or other toxins.

If you notice any sudden or unexplained skin issues, it may be time to evaluate liver health as a potential cause.

Digestive Problems

Digestive issues like nausea, indigestion, and bloating are also common indicators of liver problems. The liver produces bile, a substance essential for breaking down fats during digestion. When the liver is damaged, bile production can become insufficient, leading to undigested fat in the digestive system. This can result in bloating, cramps, and discomfort after meals.

In addition, the buildup of toxins in the bloodstream can impair the digestive system's function, leading to nausea, constipation, or diarrhea. If these digestive symptoms persist, especially when combined with other symptoms of liver dysfunction, seeking medical advice is crucial.

Jaundice: Yellowing of Skin and Eyes

Jaundice is one of the clearest signs of liver dysfunction. It is characterized by a yellowish tint in the skin, eyes, and mucous membranes. Jaundice occurs when there is an accumulation of bilirubin, a yellow pigment that the liver normally filters out from the bloodstream. When the liver becomes compromised, it struggles to process bilirubin effectively, leading to a buildup that results in yellowing.

Jaundice can be caused by several liver-related conditions, including hepatitis, cirrhosis, and liver cancer. If you notice that the whites of your eyes or your skin are turning yellow, it's important to consult a healthcare provider immediately. Jaundice may indicate a severe liver issue that requires prompt attention.

Abdominal Pain and Bloating

Abdominal pain, particularly in the upper right quadrant of the abdomen, is a common symptom of liver disease. The liver is located on the right side of the body, just beneath the rib cage, and any swelling or inflammation can cause discomfort in this area. The pain may range from a dull ache to sharp, severe discomfort, and it may be constant or come and go.

Alongside abdominal pain, bloating is another symptom to watch out for. Bloating occurs when there is an excessive buildup of gas in the stomach and intestines. In the case of liver disease, bloating can result from the liver's inability to process and eliminate toxins properly. The feeling of fullness after eating may also be present, and you may experience difficulty passing gas.

Recognizing the signs and symptoms of a compromised liver is essential for taking early action to protect your health. If you experience persistent fatigue, unexplained skin issues, digestive problems, jaundice, abdominal pain, or bloating, it's crucial to seek professional medical advice promptly. The liver is a vital organ, and catching liver issues early can make a significant difference in the effectiveness of treatment.

By understanding and identifying these warning signs, you can take the necessary steps to maintain your liver health and prevent further complications. If you suspect liver problems, don't hesitate to consult with a healthcare provider who can guide you through the appropriate tests, diagnoses, and treatments. Early intervention is key to managing liver health effectively.

How to Recognize the Warning Signs of Liver Damage

The liver, one of the most vital organs in our body, plays a crucial role in filtering toxins, storing nutrients, and supporting digestion. Despite its importance, liver damage can be a silent and gradual process, often without obvious symptoms until it has reached an advanced stage. This makes it especially important to recognize the early warning signs of liver damage. Let's explore how to identify them.

1. Unexplained Fatigue

Fatigue is one of the most common signs of liver damage. When the liver becomes damaged, its ability to detoxify the body diminishes. This causes toxins to accumulate in the blood, leading to feelings of exhaustion and lack of energy. You may feel unusually tired, even after a full night's sleep, and this fatigue can often be accompanied by a sense of weakness.

2. Jaundice (Yellowing of the Skin and Eyes)

Jaundice is a classic sign of liver problems. It occurs when the liver is unable to process bilirubin, a yellow pigment found in red blood cells. When the liver is functioning properly, bilirubin is filtered out and excreted in the stool. However, if the liver is damaged, bilirubin builds up in the blood, causing the skin and the whites of the eyes to take on a yellowish hue. If you notice jaundice, it's essential to consult a healthcare professional immediately.

3. Abdominal Pain and Discomfort

Pain or discomfort in the upper right side of the abdomen, where the liver is located, can be a sign of liver problems. This pain may be dull or sharp, and it may worsen after eating or drinking, especially if you've consumed fatty or heavy foods. In advanced liver disease, you may also experience tenderness when gently pressing on this area.

4. Nausea and Vomiting

Chronic nausea or vomiting without any clear cause could be a warning sign of liver damage. As the liver becomes overwhelmed with toxins, it can lead to digestive disturbances. The liver's inability to process and eliminate waste products can cause nausea, leading to frequent vomiting, particularly after meals.

5. Swelling in the Abdomen and Legs

The liver helps regulate fluid balance in the body. If it becomes damaged, fluid can accumulate in the abdomen (ascites) and legs (edema), leading to swelling. The swelling may be noticeable after eating, and you may feel bloated or uncomfortable. This symptom is often associated with advanced liver disease, such as cirrhosis.

6. Dark Urine and Pale Stool

Changes in urine and stool color are common indicators of liver problems. Dark urine, resembling tea or cola, can be a sign of excess bilirubin in the blood, a result of the liver's inability to process it. Pale or clay-colored stools, on the other hand, may indicate a lack of bile in the digestive system, suggesting a problem with bile production or flow due to liver damage.

7. Skin Changes and Itching

Liver damage can cause skin changes, such as rashes, redness, or darkening of the skin in certain areas (known as "spider veins"). You may also experience severe itching (pruritus), which occurs when bile acids build up in the bloodstream and are deposited in the skin. This is a common issue in individuals with liver diseases like cirrhosis or hepatitis.

8. Mental Confusion and Memory Problems

In severe cases of liver damage, such as cirrhosis, toxins that are normally filtered by the liver can accumulate in the brain. This condition, called hepatic encephalopathy, can cause confusion, memory problems, difficulty concentrating, and a general decline in mental function. If you or a loved one notice sudden changes in mental clarity, it's crucial to seek medical attention right away.

9. Easy Bruising or Bleeding

The liver is responsible for producing proteins that help with blood clotting. When liver function declines, the production of these proteins can be impaired, leading to easy bruising or spontaneous bleeding. Small cuts may take longer to stop bleeding, and you may notice bruises forming even without trauma.

Blood Sugar Fluctuations and Diabetes Symptoms

Blood sugar fluctuations are a common concern for many individuals, and they can be indicative of liver issues or a precursor to diabetes. The liver plays a central role in regulating blood sugar levels. It helps store glucose in the form of glycogen and releases it into the bloodstream when needed. If the liver is not functioning properly, it can lead to significant fluctuations in blood sugar levels, which can cause symptoms associated with both low and high blood sugar.

1. Increased Thirst and Frequent Urination

When blood sugar levels rise too high (a condition known as hyperglycemia), the kidneys work overtime to eliminate the excess sugar from the bloodstream. This leads to increased thirst (polydipsia) and frequent urination (polyuria). If you find yourself constantly thirsty and running to the bathroom, it could be a sign of high blood sugar, often linked to liver issues and diabetes.

2. Unexplained Weight Loss

Unexplained weight loss can occur when the body is unable to properly process glucose due to liver dysfunction or insulin resistance. As the body struggles to convert glucose into energy, it may start breaking down fat and muscle for fuel, leading to unintended weight loss. If you notice this symptom along with other signs of liver problems, it's crucial to consult with a healthcare professional.

3. Blurred Vision

High blood sugar levels can cause the lenses of the eyes to swell, leading to blurred vision. If you experience sudden changes in your vision, especially alongside other diabetes symptoms like fatigue, excessive thirst, and frequent urination, it could be a sign of poorly controlled blood sugar, which is often related to liver health.

4. Increased Fatigue

Fatigue is a common symptom of both high and low blood sugar. When blood sugar is too high, the body is unable to efficiently use glucose for energy. On the other hand, low blood sugar (hypoglycemia) can cause dizziness, weakness, and a feeling of extreme tiredness. Both conditions can be linked to liver dysfunction, as the liver regulates glucose release into the bloodstream.

5. Difficulty Healing and Infections

High blood sugar levels weaken the immune system and reduce the body's ability to heal wounds. If you notice that minor cuts or bruises are taking longer than usual to heal, it may be due to high blood sugar. Chronic infections, especially skin and urinary tract infections, are also more common in individuals with diabetes, which can be exacerbated by liver damage.

6. Sudden Hunger or Cravings for Sweets

Fluctuating blood sugar levels can lead to intense cravings for sugary foods. These cravings are your body's attempt to quickly raise blood sugar levels, especially when they dip too low. If you experience sudden, uncontrollable hunger or a desire for sweets, it might indicate issues with blood sugar regulation, which is often tied to liver function and insulin resistance.

Swelling in the Legs, Ankles, and Abdomen

Swelling, known medically as edema, is often an indication that something is wrong with the body's fluid balance or circulation. Swelling in the legs, ankles, and abdomen is particularly common in individuals with liver damage. The liver plays a vital role in maintaining proper fluid balance, and when it is damaged, fluid can build up in various parts of the body.

1. Fluid Retention

The liver helps produce albumin, a protein that helps maintain the body's fluid balance by preventing excessive fluid from leaking out of the blood vessels. When the liver is damaged, albumin production decreases, and fluid can escape into the surrounding tissues. This results in swelling in the legs, ankles, and abdomen. If you notice persistent swelling in these areas, it could be a sign of liver damage.

2. Ascites (Abdominal Swelling)

Ascites refers to the accumulation of fluid in the abdominal cavity, which can cause noticeable bloating and discomfort. It is commonly seen in advanced liver disease, such as cirrhosis. As the liver becomes scarred and loses its ability to function, it can lead to fluid buildup in the abdomen, resulting in painful bloating and difficulty breathing.

3. Edema in the Legs and Ankles

Swelling in the legs and ankles is another sign of fluid retention due to liver dysfunction. The liver's inability to produce enough albumin causes fluid to pool in the lower extremities, leading to noticeable swelling. This is often worse in the evening or after standing for prolonged periods.

Unexplained Weight Gain or Loss

Unexplained weight changes can be alarming and may signal an underlying health issue, including liver problems. Both weight gain and weight loss can occur in the context of liver disease, and each should be taken seriously.

1. Weight Gain Due to Fluid Retention

In cases of liver disease, particularly cirrhosis, fluid retention can cause a significant increase in weight. This weight gain is often concentrated around the abdomen and legs due to ascites and edema. While the weight gain may seem sudden and unrelated to eating habits, it's actually the result of the body's inability to maintain fluid balance.

2. Unexplained Weight Loss

On the other hand, weight loss can occur when the liver is unable to store and release energy efficiently. If the liver can't process nutrients properly, the body may turn to its fat reserves, leading to weight loss. This is often a sign of advanced liver disease, where the liver is unable to carry out its normal functions, including processing glucose and storing fat.

When to Seek Medical Help

Your liver, often called the body's unsung hero, is responsible for performing a range of vital functions that keep you healthy. While the liver is quite resilient and capable of handling a lot, it is also susceptible to damage over time, often due to lifestyle choices, environmental factors, or certain health conditions. Knowing when to seek medical help for liver-related issues is crucial, as early detection can significantly improve treatment outcomes.

Many people, unfortunately, wait too long before they seek help, thinking symptoms are temporary or not realizing that their liver health is in jeopardy. Here's what you should know about when to seek medical help if you suspect liver issues.

Recognizing the Signs of Liver Distress

The liver is a large, vital organ located in the upper right side of your abdomen. It plays a major role in detoxifying the body, producing bile for digestion, metabolizing nutrients, storing essential vitamins and minerals, and maintaining overall bodily health. When something goes wrong with your liver, it can show in various ways. Common warning signs that should not be ignored include:

1. **Fatigue and Weakness:** If you're feeling unusually tired, weak, or drained despite getting enough sleep and rest, it could be a sign of liver dysfunction. The liver is responsible for a wide variety of metabolic processes, and any imbalance in its function can make you feel tired all the time.

2. **Jaundice (Yellowing of the Skin or Eyes):** Jaundice is one of the most telling signs of liver trouble. It happens when

the liver cannot properly process bilirubin, a waste product from red blood cells. When bilirubin builds up, it can cause a yellowish tint to the skin and eyes. This is a sign that the liver might be struggling with processing waste products.

3. **Abdominal Pain and Swelling:** A swollen or painful abdomen, especially in the upper right side where the liver is located, is a common sign of liver distress. The swelling could be due to an enlarged liver (hepatomegaly) or fluid accumulation in the abdomen (ascites). These symptoms should never be overlooked, as they could indicate liver disease or cirrhosis.

4. **Nausea and Vomiting:** Persistent nausea, vomiting, or a general feeling of unwellness can be early signs of liver trouble. If you experience these symptoms alongside other liver-related issues like jaundice or abdominal pain, it's a signal to seek immediate medical attention.

5. **Changes in Urine and Stool Color:** Dark urine and pale-colored stools can indicate a liver problem. When the liver is not functioning properly, bile can back up in the body, which changes the color of urine and stool. Dark urine is typically caused by excess bilirubin being excreted in the urine, while pale stools may indicate a lack of bile in the digestive system.

6. **Unexplained Weight Loss or Loss of Appetite:** The liver plays an important role in digestion and nutrient absorption. When liver function is compromised, you might experience sudden, unexplained weight loss or a complete lack of appetite. These symptoms should prompt a visit to your healthcare provider.

When to See a Doctor

If you experience any of the above symptoms, it's important to consult a doctor without delay. While the symptoms may also be indicative of other health issues, they could be signs of liver disease or a related condition, and early intervention is key to effective treatment.

A healthcare provider will be able to evaluate your symptoms and medical history, and based on the severity and type of symptoms, they will recommend appropriate steps for further examination. In some cases, if you are at higher risk for liver disease due to factors like a history of heavy alcohol use, obesity, or hepatitis, it's advisable to consult a doctor even if you are not experiencing any symptoms.

Knowing When It's Time to Consult a Doctor

It's important to understand that not every sign of liver trouble is immediately alarming, but waiting too long to seek medical help can lead to complications. Recognizing when it's time to consult a doctor can save you a lot of worry and, in some cases, be life-saving. Below are some situations where seeing a doctor promptly is crucial:

1. You Have a Family History of Liver Disease

If liver disease runs in your family, you are at a higher risk of developing similar problems. Conditions like hereditary liver disorders (e.g., hemochromatosis, Wilson's disease) or cirrhosis due to alcohol abuse can affect more than one family member. If you have a family history of liver disease and experience any of the symptoms mentioned earlier, it's a good idea to consult a doctor right away. Your doctor may recommend regular checkups or liver function tests to detect potential problems early.

2. You Are Experiencing Severe Pain or Discomfort

Any sharp or severe pain in the upper right side of your abdomen, where the liver is located, should prompt an immediate visit to your healthcare provider. Such pain could indicate something as simple as a liver infection or inflammation, or it could be a sign of more serious conditions, such as gallstones, cirrhosis, or even liver cancer.

3. Your Liver-Related Symptoms Are Worsening

If you notice that your symptoms are progressively getting worse over time—whether it's an increase in fatigue, pain, jaundice, or swelling—it's critical to seek medical help. Worsening symptoms indicate that your liver condition may be progressing and needs immediate medical attention. Timely treatment could help manage the situation before it becomes a critical issue.

4. You Have Risk Factors for Liver Disease

Certain lifestyle choices and conditions can increase the risk of liver disease. If you're overweight, consume alcohol regularly, or have diabetes, hepatitis, or high cholesterol, you are at a higher risk. If you fall into these categories and notice even mild symptoms of liver dysfunction, it's essential to see a doctor as soon as possible. Early intervention can help prevent further liver damage and complications.

5. You Have a History of Hepatitis or Liver Injury

If you have previously been diagnosed with hepatitis or have had liver injury in the past, ongoing monitoring is important. Even if you don't currently have symptoms, your liver could still be at risk for complications like cirrhosis or liver cancer. Your doctor may recommend blood tests or imaging to monitor liver function regularly.

Diagnostic Tests: Blood Work, Ultrasounds, and More

Once you've decided to seek medical help for potential liver issues, your doctor will perform several diagnostic tests to confirm the problem and understand its severity. These tests are critical in determining the cause and extent of liver damage, and they help guide treatment options. Let's look at the most common diagnostic tests used to evaluate liver health:

1. Blood Tests (Liver Function Tests)

Blood tests are often the first step in evaluating liver health. These tests measure the levels of enzymes, proteins, and substances that the liver produces or breaks down. The most common blood tests for liver health include:

- **Alanine aminotransferase (ALT):** This enzyme is released into the blood when liver cells are damaged. Elevated ALT levels can indicate liver inflammation or damage.
- **Aspartate aminotransferase (AST):** AST is another enzyme released by the liver when it is injured. High AST levels may indicate liver disease, but AST is also present in other organs like the heart, so further testing is needed.
- **Alkaline Phosphatase (ALP):** High levels of ALP can indicate bile duct problems or liver conditions such as cirrhosis.

- **Bilirubin:** A waste product from the breakdown of red blood cells. Elevated bilirubin levels can cause jaundice and suggest liver dysfunction.
- **Albumin and Total Protein:** These proteins are made by the liver, and low levels can indicate that the liver is not functioning properly.
- **Prothrombin Time (PT):** This test measures the blood's ability to clot. A prolonged PT can indicate liver damage since the liver produces clotting factors.

2. Imaging Tests

Imaging tests are used to visualize the liver and detect structural abnormalities, such as liver enlargement, fatty liver, or tumors. Common imaging tests include:

- **Ultrasound:** A non-invasive procedure that uses sound waves to create an image of the liver. It can detect liver enlargement, fatty deposits, and other abnormalities. This is often the first imaging test used to evaluate liver health.
- **CT Scan (Computed Tomography):** This test uses X-rays to create detailed cross-sectional images of the liver. It's used to assess liver damage, tumors, or cirrhosis.
- **MRI (Magnetic Resonance Imaging):** MRI scans provide highly detailed images of the liver. They are often used to identify liver tumors, fibrosis, and cirrhosis, or when a CT scan is inconclusive.

3. Liver Biopsy

In some cases, your doctor may recommend a liver biopsy to obtain a small sample of liver tissue for analysis. This can help confirm the presence of liver disease and determine its severity, especially when imaging and blood tests are inconclusive. A biopsy is typically used in cases of chronic liver disease, cirrhosis, or unexplained liver abnormalities.

4. Elastography (FibroScan)

This is a non-invasive method used to measure the stiffness of the liver. It is often used to assess the degree of fibrosis (scarring) in the liver. A healthy liver is flexible, while a liver affected by conditions like fatty liver disease or cirrhosis becomes stiffer. This test is quick, painless, and doesn't require a needle.

Early detection of liver disease is vital to ensure the best possible outcomes, and knowing when to seek medical help is crucial. If you experience any concerning symptoms related to your liver, don't hesitate to consult a doctor. Additionally, diagnostic tests such as blood work, ultrasounds, and biopsies play a critical role in diagnosing liver conditions and determining the best treatment path. With timely medical intervention, most liver conditions can be managed effectively, so it's important to listen to your body and take action when necessary.

Chapter 4: The Science Behind Liver Detox and Regeneration

The liver is truly a marvel of biological engineering, functioning as the body's primary detoxification center. Whether we're exposed to environmental toxins, pollutants, or the natural byproducts of digestion and metabolism, the liver takes on the challenging task of neutralizing and removing harmful substances. Its capacity to regenerate itself is equally impressive, offering hope to those who suffer from liver damage.

To understand how the liver works its magic, we need to explore its mechanisms for detoxification and regeneration, as well as the various phases involved in processing the multitude of substances that enter our bodies.

How the Liver Detoxifies the Body

The liver detoxifies the body through a sophisticated, multi-step process designed to neutralize, break down, and eliminate toxins. These toxins may include alcohol, chemicals from food, environmental pollutants, pharmaceutical drugs, or even byproducts created by the body's own metabolic processes. The liver is well-equipped to handle these substances through various enzymatic processes, filtration systems, and regenerative capacities.

The detoxification process begins as blood carrying toxins enters the liver from the digestive tract and spleen. From there, the liver cells (hepatocytes) spring into action. Within the hepatocytes, enzymes and other compounds work to break down harmful substances and convert them into forms that can be safely excreted. This breakdown typically occurs in two major phases: Phase I and Phase II detoxification.

The liver also plays a key role in regulating fat and carbohydrate metabolism, helping to break down waste products from these processes, and ensuring the body remains balanced and healthy. Beyond processing toxins, the liver synthesizes proteins, produces bile (which helps digest fats), and stores important nutrients, making it an essential organ for overall well-being.

The Liver's Role in Metabolizing Toxins

Every day, the liver is exposed to an array of toxins, from the chemicals in food and beverages to pollution and medications. The liver metabolizes these toxins using a system of enzymes designed to neutralize them, converting them into less harmful substances. This is a delicate, well-orchestrated process that involves both Phase I and Phase II detoxification systems.

- **Phase I Detoxification (Cytochrome P450 Enzymes)**: During Phase I, enzymes, primarily in the cytochrome P450 family, break down toxins into intermediate metabolites. These enzymes can be thought of as the liver's "first responders," ready to attack harmful chemicals. Some of these metabolites, however, are still reactive and may cause damage if not processed in Phase II. These reactive intermediates can also be harmful if they're not efficiently neutralized.

- **Phase II Detoxification (Conjugation Reactions)**: Phase II detoxification is crucial because it converts these reactive metabolites from Phase I into water-soluble compounds that can be excreted through the urine or bile. This process involves conjugation reactions where molecules like glutathione, sulfur, or amino acids are added to the intermediate metabolites, rendering them less toxic.

As a result, the liver is highly effective at metabolizing and neutralizing a wide range of substances, transforming them into forms that can either be excreted via the kidneys or sent into the bile for elimination in the stool.

But detoxification doesn't stop there. The liver also plays a role in regenerating itself to maintain its function and resilience over time.

Phases of Detoxification and Their Importance

Detoxification in the liver occurs in two main phases, each vital to ensuring that toxins are properly neutralized and eliminated. These phases work in tandem to protect the body from the harmful effects of the toxins we encounter every day.

Phase I: Oxidation, Reduction, and Hydrolysis

Phase I detoxification primarily involves oxidation, reduction, and hydrolysis reactions. In this phase, enzymes like cytochrome P450 break down toxins by adding oxygen atoms to their molecular structure, making them easier to process. However, this process can sometimes produce free radicals or reactive intermediates, which are unstable molecules that can damage healthy cells and tissues. The body must quickly neutralize these reactive intermediates to prevent harm.

For example, alcohol and certain prescription medications are broken down in Phase I through the cytochrome P450 enzymes. These processes help transform harmful substances into more manageable compounds for Phase II.

Why is Phase I important?
Phase I is essential because it activates toxins, preparing them for the conjugation process in Phase II. However, it's crucial that Phase

I doesn't run too quickly, as the buildup of free radicals and reactive intermediates can cause oxidative stress, leading to inflammation and cellular damage. This is why supporting Phase II detoxification is equally important.

Phase II: Conjugation and Elimination

Once the liver has broken down toxins in Phase I, the next step is to conjugate these molecules to make them water-soluble and easier to eliminate from the body. Phase II detoxification reactions involve adding specific molecules, such as glutathione, sulfur, or glucuronic acid, to the reactive intermediates created in Phase I. These conjugates are less toxic and can now be safely excreted via the kidneys or intestines.

Why is Phase II important?

Phase II detoxification is crucial because it helps ensure that the byproducts created in Phase I do not remain in their harmful forms. If Phase II is impaired or slow, reactive metabolites can accumulate, increasing the risk of liver damage, inflammation, and other health problems. Many lifestyle factors, such as poor diet, stress, and lack of exercise, can impair Phase II detoxification, underscoring the importance of liver health maintenance.

Liver Regeneration: How the Liver Heals Itself

One of the most extraordinary features of the liver is its ability to regenerate after injury or damage. Unlike many other organs, the liver can regrow lost tissue and resume its normal functions. This regeneration process is vital for maintaining health and ensuring that the body can continue to detoxify and process nutrients efficiently.

The Mechanisms of Liver Regeneration

The liver's regenerative capacity is powered by hepatocytes (liver cells). When liver tissue is damaged, these cells begin to proliferate, creating new liver cells to replace the damaged ones. This regeneration can occur even in the presence of chronic liver disease, such as fatty liver disease or cirrhosis, although regeneration is less effective when the damage is extensive.

Liver regeneration is influenced by several factors:

1. **Growth Factors**: Molecules such as hepatocyte growth factor (HGF) and epidermal growth factor (EGF) play key roles in stimulating liver cell proliferation and tissue repair.
2. **Stem Cells**: The liver contains a small population of progenitor or stem cells that can differentiate into hepatocytes and other liver cell types when needed.
3. **Nutrient and Hormonal Signals**: Nutritional factors, including vitamins, minerals, and amino acids, help support liver regeneration. Hormones like insulin and thyroid hormones also play essential roles in the process.

Although the liver can regenerate effectively, chronic damage from factors such as alcohol abuse, viral infections (hepatitis), or an unhealthy diet can impair its regenerative capacity. This is why it is essential to maintain liver health through proper diet, exercise, and lifestyle changes.

Support for Liver Detox and Regeneration

To optimize the liver's detoxification and regeneration abilities, it's important to focus on providing the liver with the right nutrients, exercise, and overall care. A well-balanced diet rich in antioxidants, healthy fats, and anti-inflammatory compounds can support both detoxification and liver repair.

- **Support for Phase I and Phase II Detoxification**: Certain nutrients, such as B-vitamins, vitamin C, and sulfur-containing compounds (like garlic and onions), can support the liver's enzymatic detox processes.
- **Anti-inflammatory Foods**: Foods such as turmeric, green tea, and omega-3-rich foods can help reduce inflammation in the liver and support the regenerative process.
- **Hydration**: Staying hydrated is crucial to support the liver's detoxification processes, as it helps flush toxins from the body through the kidneys and digestive system.

Liver Regeneration: Can the Liver Heal Itself?

The liver is the body's most extraordinary organ when it comes to healing and regeneration. It has a remarkable ability to repair itself, often recovering from damage that would be impossible for most other organs. However, the liver's ability to regenerate is not limitless. Understanding how it works can help us appreciate its role in overall health and how we can best support it for optimal function.

The liver is unique because it can regenerate from a variety of injuries, including damage from toxins, viruses, and certain diseases. This regenerative ability is one of the reasons that many people don't realize they have liver problems until it's too late. The liver has a backup plan. It can grow new cells to replace damaged ones, effectively making it the body's self-healing powerhouse.

But while regeneration is possible, it is not an indefinite process. The liver can only regenerate to a certain point before it reaches a stage where the damage is irreversible. This is why liver health is so important, as taking steps to protect it early on can prevent long-term damage.

The Liver's Unique Ability to Regenerate

The liver's regenerative power is so impressive that it can regrow up to 70% of its original mass after surgical removal, as long as the remaining liver tissue is healthy. This capacity for regeneration is driven by the liver cells known as hepatocytes. When the liver is damaged, hepatocytes are stimulated to divide and form new cells. This process is known as *regeneration*.

One of the key reasons why the liver has this ability lies in its cellular structure. Unlike most organs in the body, which consist of specialized cells that perform specific functions, the liver has a large number of unspecialized cells that can adapt to many different functions. These cells can regenerate even in the presence of damage.

For example, if a person suffers from a liver injury due to alcohol abuse or a viral infection, the liver can attempt to heal itself through the rapid production of new hepatocytes. Even if a portion of the liver is removed, as long as the remaining liver tissue is healthy, it can grow back.

Interestingly, the liver doesn't necessarily have to grow back to its exact original shape and size. What's important is that it regains its full function. The liver is responsible for numerous vital functions, including detoxifying the blood, producing bile for digestion, storing glycogen for energy, and synthesizing proteins. As long as these functions can be restored, the liver has done its job.

But what exactly triggers the regeneration process? When liver cells are damaged or destroyed, a series of signaling molecules are released. These molecules activate the remaining healthy liver cells to begin the regeneration process. This complex biochemical process ensures that the liver remains functional even as it heals itself.

How to Support the Liver's Natural Healing Process

If you want to give your liver the best chance to heal and regenerate, there are several key steps you can take to support its natural healing process. The liver can't regenerate without the right conditions, and your lifestyle choices play a large role in making those conditions optimal.

1. **Proper Nutrition:** Eating a well-balanced diet is one of the most important factors in supporting liver regeneration. Nutrients like antioxidants, vitamins, and minerals are essential for liver repair. Foods rich in vitamin C, vitamin E, zinc, and selenium help reduce inflammation and support the liver in its detoxification process.

   Foods to Include in Your Diet:

   - Leafy greens, such as spinach and kale, are high in antioxidants and promote liver detoxification.
   - Fatty fish like salmon and mackerel are rich in omega-3 fatty acids, which help reduce liver inflammation.
   - Garlic and onions contain sulfur compounds that assist in detoxification and support liver health.
   - Turmeric contains curcumin, a compound known for its anti-inflammatory properties that can help with liver healing.

2. **Avoid Toxins:** The liver plays a key role in detoxifying the body. When toxins build up in the liver, it can impair its

ability to regenerate. It's essential to avoid alcohol, tobacco, and other harmful substances that can overload the liver.

Reducing your exposure to environmental toxins, such as pesticides, industrial chemicals, and pollution, is also crucial. These toxins can disrupt the liver's ability to repair itself, leading to chronic damage.

3. **Regular Exercise:** Physical activity helps improve circulation and promotes overall metabolic health. It's important to maintain a healthy weight, as obesity is one of the major contributors to fatty liver disease. Regular exercise also supports the liver by reducing inflammation, improving insulin sensitivity, and promoting healthy fat metabolism.

Aim for at least 30 minutes of moderate exercise, such as walking, swimming, or cycling, five days a week. This will not only help with liver regeneration but also improve your overall health.

4. **Hydration:** Drinking enough water is vital for liver function. Staying hydrated ensures that the liver can flush out toxins effectively. Aim for at least 8 cups of water a day, and avoid sugary drinks or excessive amounts of caffeine that can strain the liver.

5. **Stress Management:** Chronic stress is another factor that can negatively impact liver health. When you're stressed, your body produces more cortisol, a hormone that can contribute to liver damage if levels remain elevated over time. Techniques such as meditation, deep breathing, yoga, and mindfulness can help reduce stress and promote a

healthy liver.

Factors That Hinder Liver Regeneration

While the liver has an extraordinary ability to regenerate, there are several factors that can hinder or even stop this process. Chronic damage, poor lifestyle choices, and certain health conditions can overwhelm the liver's regenerative capacity. Recognizing these factors can help you take steps to prevent them from limiting your liver's ability to heal.

1. **Chronic Alcohol Consumption:** Alcohol is one of the leading causes of liver damage. Over time, excessive drinking can cause alcoholic liver disease (ALD), which can lead to cirrhosis and liver failure. Chronic alcohol consumption impairs the liver's ability to regenerate, as it continually overworks the organ and causes inflammation. The liver's cells become damaged, and regeneration becomes less efficient with each drink.

2. **Fatty Liver Disease:** Non-alcoholic fatty liver disease (NAFLD) and alcoholic fatty liver disease (AFLD) are both conditions where fat accumulates in the liver, impairing its function. If left untreated, fatty liver can lead to cirrhosis and liver failure. In the early stages, fatty liver can often be reversed with changes in diet and lifestyle, but in the later stages, the liver's regenerative capacity can become severely diminished.

3. **Chronic Hepatitis Infections:** Hepatitis B and C are viral infections that cause inflammation in the liver. Over time, this inflammation can result in scarring (cirrhosis) and liver cancer. Although the liver can regenerate to some extent

after viral infections, prolonged inflammation from chronic hepatitis can overwhelm the liver's healing abilities, leading to irreversible damage.

4. **Obesity:** Obesity is a major risk factor for liver disease, including fatty liver, cirrhosis, and liver cancer. Excess fat in the liver can create inflammation, which makes it difficult for the liver to regenerate. Additionally, obesity can contribute to insulin resistance, which worsens liver damage. Maintaining a healthy weight is essential for supporting liver health and regeneration.

5. **Toxin Overload:** Chronic exposure to toxins such as environmental pollutants, medications, and recreational drugs can overwhelm the liver's ability to detoxify the body. Over time, this reduces the liver's capacity to regenerate, leading to liver damage. Even common medications, such as acetaminophen (Tylenol), can harm the liver if taken in excess, so it's important to be mindful of the medications you take.

6. **Genetic Factors:** Certain genetic conditions, such as Wilson's disease or hemochromatosis, affect the liver's ability to function properly. These inherited conditions can result in abnormal accumulation of copper or iron in the liver, leading to damage and scarring. In these cases, the liver may still regenerate to some extent, but the underlying genetic issue must be addressed to avoid long-term damage.

7. **Aging:** As we age, the liver's ability to regenerate naturally declines. Older individuals may find that their liver takes longer to heal from damage or injury. This is one reason why it's so important to adopt healthy lifestyle habits early

in life to protect the liver from unnecessary wear and tear.

The liver is truly a marvel of nature. Its ability to regenerate after injury or damage is a testament to the body's resilience. However, it is important to remember that the liver's regenerative capacity has limits, and factors like alcohol consumption, obesity, and chronic diseases can hinder this process. By adopting a healthy lifestyle—through proper nutrition, regular exercise, hydration, and stress management—you can support your liver's natural healing process and ensure its health for years to come.

Understanding the liver's regenerative ability gives us a valuable tool in preventing liver disease. We must do our part to protect this powerful organ, enabling it to continue doing its vital work in the body. By taking action now, we can help maintain liver health and enjoy a better quality of life.

The Importance of Liver Health for Long-Term Wellness

The liver is one of the most vital organs in the body. Yet, it is often the most overlooked when it comes to health discussions. Situated in the upper right side of the abdomen, the liver is a multi-functional organ responsible for a wide range of processes essential to keeping the body running smoothly. Understanding the role of the liver and how crucial it is for overall wellness is key to maintaining long-term health.

The Vital Functions of the Liver

At a basic level, the liver serves as a detoxification powerhouse. It processes harmful substances, such as toxins, drugs, and alcohol, turning them into waste products that can be safely eliminated from the body. Without a functioning liver, these harmful substances would build up in the bloodstream, potentially leading to life-threatening conditions.

But detoxification is just the beginning. The liver is involved in over 500 other vital functions. It helps regulate blood sugar levels, stores and releases energy, and produces important proteins like albumin, which keeps fluid in the bloodstream and supports proper circulation. The liver also plays a significant role in digestion by producing bile, which is essential for breaking down fats in food.

This organ also manages fat and cholesterol levels, converting excess sugars and fats into a form that the body can use later. Furthermore, the liver is a key player in the body's immune system, filtering out pathogens and bacteria from the blood. This broad spectrum of duties highlights why liver health is so crucial for overall well-being.

Why Liver Health Matters Long-Term

As we age, the importance of liver health becomes more evident. Many of the body's vital processes depend on the liver functioning optimally. For instance, without sufficient bile production, you can experience digestive issues, leading to bloating, discomfort, and malnutrition over time. If liver function becomes impaired, it can lead to a host of long-term complications such as liver disease, cirrhosis, and liver failure, each of which can significantly reduce quality of life.

Maintaining a healthy liver throughout life allows you to stay active, energized, and free from chronic conditions. This makes liver health central to long-term wellness. By supporting your liver with a balanced diet, regular exercise, and avoiding harmful substances, you ensure the organ can continue to perform its crucial functions for years to come.

Liver Health and Aging

As we get older, our liver's ability to regenerate naturally declines. It becomes less efficient at filtering toxins, producing essential proteins, and storing nutrients. The effects of this gradual decline can go unnoticed at first, but over time, they can add up, leading to chronic diseases or even liver failure if not properly managed. This is why prioritizing liver health is especially critical as you age.

How Liver Health Affects Your Immune System

The liver is not only an organ for detoxification but also an integral part of the body's immune system. You might be surprised to learn that the liver serves as one of the body's largest immune organs. It helps fight infections, manage inflammation, and protect against harmful invaders like bacteria and viruses. Therefore, liver health directly impacts how well your body can defend itself from illness and maintain a strong immune system.

The Role of the Liver in Immunity

The liver contains special immune cells called Kupffer cells. These cells act as the first line of defense against bacteria, viruses, and other pathogens in the blood. Kupffer cells identify these harmful invaders and help eliminate them before they can cause damage. Additionally, the liver plays a role in producing certain proteins, including C-reactive protein (CRP), which helps to regulate inflammation in the body.

When the liver is compromised, its ability to fight off infections and regulate immune responses diminishes. As a result, people with liver conditions like cirrhosis, fatty liver disease, or hepatitis are at a higher risk of developing infections, as their immune systems become weaker and less effective. This creates a vicious cycle where liver damage weakens immunity, and a weakened immune system makes it harder for the liver to heal.

Liver Disease and Immunodeficiency

Chronic liver diseases, such as cirrhosis or hepatitis, can severely impair immune function. In these cases, the liver's ability to produce key immune components, such as antibodies and cytokines, is reduced. This makes it harder for the body to respond to infections. Additionally, toxins that the liver normally filters from the bloodstream may build up, causing an inflammatory response that further weakens the immune system.

People with compromised liver function may also experience autoimmune disorders, where the immune system mistakenly attacks the body's own tissues. This can result in additional strain on the liver, further diminishing its effectiveness in fighting infections and managing inflammation.

Strengthening Immunity Through Liver Health

Maintaining a healthy liver ensures that it can support a strong immune system. By eating a nutrient-rich diet, staying hydrated, and avoiding excessive alcohol or harmful toxins, you help your liver work effectively to protect you from disease. Regular exercise can also reduce inflammation, boost circulation, and support liver function, further enhancing immune system health.

Connection Between Liver Function and Mental Clarity

You might not immediately think of the liver when considering mental clarity or cognitive function, but the connection between liver health and brain function is profound. A properly functioning liver ensures that the brain has access to the necessary nutrients and a clean environment to operate at its best. Conversely, liver dysfunction can have a negative impact on mental clarity, leading to brain fog, fatigue, and even more serious cognitive issues.

How the Liver Supports Brain Function

The liver performs many critical tasks that directly support brain health. One of its most important roles is the removal of toxic substances from the bloodstream. Without the liver filtering out toxins such as ammonia, these harmful substances can accumulate in the body and reach the brain, potentially causing confusion, forgetfulness, or difficulty concentrating. High levels of ammonia, for instance, are often associated with hepatic encephalopathy, a condition that can occur when the liver is unable to detoxify the body properly.

Furthermore, the liver helps regulate blood sugar levels. When the liver is functioning well, it ensures a steady release of glucose into the bloodstream, providing the brain with a constant supply of energy. If the liver is struggling, blood sugar levels can become unstable, leading to symptoms such as brain fog, fatigue, and difficulty concentrating.

Liver Disease and Cognitive Decline

Liver disease can result in cognitive issues due to the buildup of toxins in the bloodstream, including in the brain. In individuals with chronic liver conditions such as cirrhosis, mental health problems like anxiety and depression are more common. This is because the liver's ability to eliminate toxins is compromised, leading to a buildup of substances that can alter brain function.

Moreover, liver disease can contribute to hormonal imbalances, which also affect cognitive function. These hormonal shifts may manifest as mood swings, irritability, and even memory problems. Maintaining liver health, therefore, is essential for protecting both mental clarity and emotional well-being.

Improving Mental Clarity Through Liver Health

To support mental clarity, it's essential to take care of your liver. Staying hydrated, eating a balanced diet rich in antioxidants and healthy fats, and managing stress are all important steps to promote liver health and improve brain function. Avoiding excessive alcohol and harmful substances also protects both your liver and your cognitive abilities.

The Link Between Liver Health and Chronic Diseases (Diabetes, Heart Disease, etc.)

Chronic diseases such as diabetes, heart disease, and even some forms of cancer are often linked to poor liver health. The liver is responsible for maintaining blood sugar levels, regulating cholesterol, and processing fats in the body—all of which are key factors in the development of chronic diseases. By understanding this connection, you can take proactive steps to support your liver and reduce your risk of these life-threatening conditions.

The Role of the Liver in Managing Blood Sugar

The liver is involved in storing and releasing glucose (sugar) into the bloodstream as needed. It helps maintain a balance in blood sugar levels by storing excess glucose as glycogen and releasing it when blood sugar levels drop. However, in individuals with poor liver function, this process may become impaired, leading to insulin resistance—a key factor in the development of type 2 diabetes.

A liver that is overwhelmed with fat, toxins, or inflammation struggles to manage blood sugar efficiently. Over time, this can lead to the development of diabetes, a chronic condition where the body becomes resistant to insulin and can no longer regulate blood sugar levels properly.

Liver Disease and Heart Health

The liver also plays a significant role in regulating cholesterol levels. It produces the lipoproteins necessary to carry cholesterol in the blood. When the liver is compromised, this balance can be disrupted, leading to high cholesterol levels, which in turn increase the risk of heart disease. A fatty liver, often caused by poor diet, excessive alcohol consumption, or obesity, can significantly raise the levels of bad cholesterol (LDL) while lowering good cholesterol (HDL), contributing to the formation of plaque in the arteries and increasing the risk of heart attacks and strokes.

Protecting Your Liver to Prevent Chronic Diseases

By maintaining liver health, you can reduce your risk of developing chronic conditions like diabetes and heart disease. Adopting a healthy diet, exercising regularly, and avoiding harmful substances such as alcohol and tobacco can significantly reduce the strain on your liver, helping to prevent the onset of these diseases. Keeping your liver healthy is an investment in preventing long-term health problems.

Chapter 5: Nutrition for Liver Health

The liver, one of the most vital organs in our body, plays a central role in detoxification, digestion, metabolism, and nutrient storage. It processes everything we eat and drink, including harmful substances like alcohol, medication, and environmental toxins. Therefore, maintaining liver health is crucial for overall well-being. A poor diet and unhealthy lifestyle choices can stress the liver and make it less effective in its essential functions.

One of the most important things you can do to protect your liver is to adopt a liver-friendly diet. Eating a balanced, nutrient-rich diet not only supports liver function but also reduces the risk of liver-related diseases such as fatty liver, cirrhosis, and hepatitis. Nutrition for liver health focuses on consuming foods that reduce inflammation, improve digestion, and assist in detoxification.

In this chapter, we will delve deeper into specific foods and nutrients that support liver health. We will also explore the importance of anti-inflammatory foods, liver-supporting vegetables, and healthy fats. These food groups have been shown to provide both immediate and long-term benefits for your liver.

Foods That Promote Liver Health

The liver is constantly working to filter toxins, process fats, and regulate essential functions in the body. Therefore, foods that enhance liver health need to be nutrient-dense, anti-inflammatory, and rich in antioxidants. Here is a comprehensive look at the foods that are particularly beneficial for the liver.

1. High-fiber foods

Fiber plays a critical role in maintaining liver health. It helps promote healthy digestion and prevents the buildup of fats in the liver. By improving digestion, fiber allows the liver to process toxins more efficiently. Foods that are rich in fiber include:

- **Whole grains**: Brown rice, quinoa, barley, and oats are excellent sources of fiber and help in liver detoxification.
- **Fruits and vegetables**: Apples, pears, berries, carrots, and sweet potatoes are packed with fiber and essential vitamins.
- **Legumes**: Beans, lentils, and chickpeas are high in fiber, which can help reduce the liver's workload.

2. Antioxidant-rich foods

Antioxidants help neutralize harmful free radicals that can damage liver cells. Antioxidant-rich foods protect the liver from oxidative stress and inflammation. Key foods that are packed with antioxidants include:

- **Berries**: Blueberries, strawberries, and blackberries are rich in antioxidants that help prevent liver damage.
- **Pomegranates**: These are particularly beneficial due to their high antioxidant content, which can help improve liver function.
- **Beets**: Known for their high fiber and antioxidant content, beets support liver detoxification and reduce oxidative stress.

3. Protein-rich foods

Liver cells need protein to regenerate and repair. Opt for high-quality sources of protein that are easily digestible, such as:

- **Fish**: Salmon, sardines, and mackerel are excellent choices because they are high in omega-3 fatty acids, which reduce inflammation in the liver.
- **Eggs**: Rich in protein, eggs provide the amino acids necessary for liver repair.
- **Poultry**: Chicken and turkey are lean protein sources that help maintain liver health.

4. Hydrating foods

The liver's detoxification processes rely on hydration. Drinking sufficient water is essential, but eating hydrating foods can also help. Water-rich foods like watermelon, cucumber, and citrus fruits provide hydration and essential vitamins for liver health.

Anti-Inflammatory Foods: Turmeric, Garlic, Green Tea

Inflammation is one of the primary contributors to liver disease. Chronic inflammation can damage liver tissue, leading to conditions like fatty liver disease and cirrhosis. Incorporating anti-inflammatory foods into your diet can help calm this internal inflammation and support liver health.

1. Turmeric

Turmeric is one of the most powerful anti-inflammatory spices in the world. The active compound, **curcumin**, has been extensively researched for its anti-inflammatory, antioxidant, and liver-protective properties. Curcumin helps reduce liver inflammation and enhances the liver's ability to detoxify. It is known to increase the production of bile, which helps the liver break down fats more efficiently.

To maximize the benefits of turmeric, try incorporating it into your daily diet. You can add turmeric to soups, smoothies, and curries or even drink a cup of turmeric tea. However, for optimal absorption, it's beneficial to combine turmeric with black pepper, as piperine (found in black pepper) enhances the absorption of curcumin by up to 2000%.

2. Garlic

Garlic has long been known for its medicinal properties, and research suggests that it plays a significant role in liver health. Garlic contains sulfur compounds that activate liver enzymes responsible for flushing out toxins. It also has potent anti-inflammatory and antioxidant properties that protect the liver from damage.

Garlic consumption has been linked to a decrease in liver fat accumulation and can aid in reducing the risk of liver disease. Whether raw or cooked, garlic can be easily added to a variety of dishes, such as stir-fries, sauces, or soups.

3. Green Tea

Green tea is another excellent anti-inflammatory food, rich in antioxidants known as **catechins**. These antioxidants have been shown to improve liver function, reduce fat buildup in the liver, and protect against oxidative stress. Drinking green tea regularly has been associated with a lower risk of liver disease and improved liver health in individuals with fatty liver disease.

For maximum benefit, aim to drink 2-3 cups of green tea a day. Try to avoid adding sugar or sweeteners, as they can negate some of the benefits of green tea.

Liver-Supporting Vegetables: Cruciferous and Leafy Greens

Certain vegetables are particularly beneficial for liver health due to their detoxifying properties and ability to support the liver's natural cleansing processes. Cruciferous and leafy greens are among the most powerful vegetables for promoting liver function.

1. Cruciferous Vegetables (Broccoli, Cauliflower, Brussels Sprouts)

Cruciferous vegetables, including broccoli, cauliflower, cabbage, and Brussels sprouts, are packed with nutrients that support liver detoxification. They contain **sulfur compounds**, which activate liver enzymes that help neutralize and eliminate toxins. These vegetables are also rich in **fiber**, which aids in digestion and prevents fatty buildup in the liver.

Broccoli, in particular, contains a compound called **sulforaphane**, which has been shown to reduce liver inflammation and improve liver function. Eating cruciferous vegetables regularly can help lower the risk of liver disease and promote overall liver health.

2. Leafy Greens (Spinach, Kale, Dandelion Greens)

Leafy greens such as spinach, kale, dandelion greens, and collard greens are rich in antioxidants, vitamins, and minerals that support liver function. They help to reduce oxidative stress, a key factor in liver damage. Additionally, leafy greens are high in **chlorophyll**, which binds to toxins and helps to eliminate them from the body, reducing the burden on the liver.

Kale, spinach, and dandelion greens also contain compounds that help increase bile production, which is essential for fat digestion and liver detoxification. These greens are easy to incorporate into smoothies, salads, and soups.

Healthy Fats: Avocados, Olive Oil, Nuts

Although fat has often been viewed as a harmful nutrient, healthy fats are essential for liver health. Healthy fats provide the necessary energy for the body, support hormone production, and aid in the absorption of fat-soluble vitamins. When choosing fats for liver health, it's important to focus on healthy fats that reduce inflammation and improve liver function.

1. Avocados

Avocados are rich in monounsaturated fats, which are known to help reduce liver fat accumulation and lower inflammation. They are also a great source of **glutathione**, a powerful antioxidant that helps detoxify the liver. The fiber content in avocados also helps in digestion and supports healthy liver function.

Research shows that consuming avocados regularly may reduce the risk of developing liver disease and improve liver health. Add avocado to salads, sandwiches, or smoothies for a nutrient-packed meal.

2. Olive Oil

Extra virgin olive oil is another excellent source of healthy fats. It contains high levels of **oleic acid**, a monounsaturated fat that has anti-inflammatory effects and may help protect the liver from damage. Olive oil is also rich in antioxidants, such as **vitamin E**, which further help reduce liver inflammation and oxidative stress.

Consuming olive oil regularly has been linked to improved liver function, especially in people with fatty liver disease. Drizzle olive oil over salads, vegetables, or use it as a cooking oil to reap its health benefits.

3. Nuts

Nuts, such as almonds, walnuts, and cashews, are rich in healthy fats, protein, and fiber. Walnuts, in particular, contain high levels of **omega-3 fatty acids**, which help reduce liver fat and inflammation. Nuts also provide essential vitamins and minerals, including **vitamin E**, which protect the liver from oxidative damage.

Including a variety of nuts in your diet can help support liver health, but it's important to eat them in moderation due to their calorie density. Add a handful of nuts to salads, yogurt, or enjoy them as a snack.

The Pro-Liver Diet: What to Eat and What to Avoid

The liver, as one of the hardest-working organs in our body, requires a well-balanced and nutrient-dense diet to function optimally. As an experienced professional in this field, I cannot emphasize enough the importance of adopting a **Pro-Liver Diet**—a way of eating that supports the liver in its role as a detoxifier, metabolizer, and a producer of critical proteins. The liver helps with digestion, produces bile, detoxifies harmful substances, and regulates blood sugar. The right foods provide essential nutrients that enhance liver function, while the wrong foods can put unnecessary stress on it.

A Pro-Liver Diet is built around whole, unprocessed foods, packed with antioxidants, vitamins, and minerals, which support liver regeneration, help reduce inflammation, and promote the detoxification process. Below, I'll guide you through what to eat, as well as foods you should avoid to keep your liver in peak condition.

What to Eat for Liver Health

1. **Leafy Greens and Cruciferous Vegetables** These vegetables are packed with fiber and essential nutrients that help promote liver detoxification. **Spinach, kale, broccoli, and Brussels sprouts** contain compounds that increase the production of enzymes responsible for detoxifying the liver. Additionally, they help reduce fat buildup, which is important for preventing fatty liver disease.

2. **Berries and Antioxidant-Rich Fruits** Berries—such as **blueberries, raspberries, and strawberries**—are rich in antioxidants that fight free radicals in the body. These fruits contain vitamins C and E, which help reduce liver inflammation and oxidative stress. Also, antioxidant-rich foods like **grapes, oranges, and apples** help keep the liver's cells healthy and protect it from further damage.

3. **Healthy Fats** The liver needs healthy fats to support its functions, but not all fats are created equal. **Omega-3 fatty acids**, found in foods like **salmon, mackerel, chia seeds, flaxseeds, and walnuts**, have anti-inflammatory effects and help protect the liver from the damaging effects of high-fat diets. **Olive oil** is another great source of healthy fats that support liver health by reducing fat buildup.

4. **Turmeric and Garlic Turmeric** is one of the most powerful natural liver protectors available. Its active compound, **curcumin**, helps reduce inflammation in the liver and supports liver cell regeneration. **Garlic**, on the

other hand, contains sulfur compounds that stimulate liver detoxification and enhance the production of liver enzymes that help cleanse the body.

5. **Whole Grains Oats, quinoa, brown rice, and whole wheat** are excellent sources of fiber, which helps the liver flush out toxins. Whole grains also help maintain a stable blood sugar level, which reduces the risk of developing liver-related conditions like fatty liver disease.

6. **Liver-Boosting Beverages** Hydration is essential for liver function. Drinking **green tea** regularly provides antioxidants and catechins, which promote liver health by boosting its natural detoxifying processes. Additionally, fresh **lemon water** aids digestion and enhances liver enzyme function.

What to Avoid for Liver Health

1. **Processed Sugar** The liver processes sugar, but excessive consumption leads to fat buildup in the liver, a condition known as **non-alcoholic fatty liver disease** (NAFLD). **Refined sugars** found in candies, sodas, baked goods, and processed foods contribute to inflammation and liver damage. Keeping your sugar intake low helps prevent the liver from becoming overwhelmed and ensures better overall liver function.

2. **Trans Fats Trans fats**, found in many processed and fried foods, are highly detrimental to liver health. These fats can cause fat to accumulate in the liver, leading to insulin resistance and fatty liver disease. **Fast food, packaged snacks**, and **margarine** are common sources of trans fats.

They should be avoided at all costs if you want to keep your liver functioning at its best.

3. **Alcohol** Excessive alcohol intake is one of the most well-known causes of liver damage. Alcohol can overwhelm the liver's detoxification processes and lead to inflammation, cirrhosis, or liver failure. While moderate drinking may be safe for some individuals, chronic alcohol consumption significantly increases the risk of liver disease. For those with existing liver conditions, abstaining from alcohol is imperative.

4. **Excessive Salt** While not as directly harmful as sugar or alcohol, too much sodium can cause fluid retention, increase blood pressure, and put stress on the liver. Foods high in sodium include canned soups, processed meats, and salty snacks. Always choose fresh, whole foods and use herbs and spices instead of salt for seasoning.

Building a Liver-Friendly Meal Plan

Creating a **Liver-Friendly Meal Plan** is a great way to ensure that your diet is tailored to support optimal liver function. A well-designed meal plan takes into account the liver's need for nutrients that promote detoxification, reduce inflammation, and prevent fat accumulation. Here's a step-by-step guide to building a meal plan that promotes liver health:

Step 1: Plan for Variety

A healthy liver thrives on variety, as different foods provide different nutrients that the liver needs to function. Incorporate a range of **fruits, vegetables, whole grains, healthy fats, and lean**

proteins into your meals. Variety ensures that your body receives all the vitamins, minerals, and antioxidants needed for detoxification and overall liver health.

Step 2: Focus on Fiber

Fiber is crucial for digestive health, and it also supports the liver in flushing out toxins. Each meal should include **fiber-rich foods** like leafy greens, fruits, and whole grains. Try including **brown rice or quinoa** in your lunch and **oats** for breakfast. This helps improve bile production, a critical function of the liver that aids digestion.

Step 3: Prioritize Lean Protein Sources

Protein helps the body repair liver cells and create enzymes that support detoxification. Opt for lean sources of protein like **chicken, turkey, fish**, or **plant-based options** like beans, lentils, and tofu. Avoid fatty cuts of meat, which can increase inflammation and contribute to fatty liver disease.

Step 4: Include Healthy Fats

Healthy fats, like **avocado, nuts, and olive oil**, should be incorporated into your meal plan to promote liver health. These fats help regulate cholesterol levels and reduce inflammation. In particular, **omega-3 fatty acids** found in oily fish and certain seeds (like chia and flax) provide excellent anti-inflammatory benefits.

Step 5: Incorporate Liver-Detoxifying Foods

Certain foods are natural liver detoxifiers. Be sure to include **garlic, turmeric, green tea, and citrus fruits** in your meal plan. These foods stimulate liver function, help reduce oxidative stress, and support the liver's ability to neutralize toxins.

Foods to Avoid: Processed Sugar, Trans Fats, and Alcohol

When crafting a liver-friendly meal plan, it's equally important to avoid foods that can overwhelm the liver's ability to detoxify the body and cause fat buildup. The three main culprits to be cautious of are **processed sugar**, **trans fats**, and **alcohol**.

Processed Sugar

Sugar is an essential part of our diet, but too much can wreak havoc on your liver. Processed sugar, particularly **fructose**, is metabolized in the liver and can contribute to fat storage, insulin resistance, and the development of fatty liver disease. Avoid sugary foods like **cakes, candies, sodas**, and **high-fructose corn syrup**, which can increase the burden on the liver. Instead, choose natural sweeteners like **honey** or **stevia** in moderation if you need to satisfy your sweet tooth.

Trans Fats

Trans fats, found in many processed foods, are known to increase fat accumulation in the liver and elevate the risk of insulin resistance and inflammation. Foods high in trans fats include **fried foods**, **store-bought pastries**, and **margarine**. Always opt for **healthy oils** such as **extra virgin olive oil** or **coconut oil** and avoid pre-packaged foods that list **partially hydrogenated oils** in their ingredients.

Alcohol

Excessive alcohol consumption is one of the leading causes of liver damage, and even moderate drinking can be harmful for those with pre-existing liver conditions. The liver metabolizes alcohol, but consuming large amounts can lead to liver inflammation, fat buildup, and cirrhosis. To protect your liver, it is best to avoid alcohol altogether or limit your intake to occasional, moderate servings.

Portion Control and Mindful Eating for Liver Health

Lastly, **portion control** and **mindful eating** are key practices for supporting liver health. The liver is designed to handle a balanced diet, but overloading it with excess food can lead to weight gain, fatty liver disease, and other metabolic disorders. Mindful eating helps you tune in to your body's hunger signals and make healthier choices for your liver.

Portion Control

Portion control is a simple yet powerful tool for maintaining liver health. Eating too much food, even if it's healthy, can strain the liver and contribute to obesity, which is a significant risk factor for liver disease. A helpful strategy is to use smaller plates, avoid second servings, and listen to your body when it signals fullness.

Mindful Eating

Mindful eating involves paying full attention to the food you are consuming—eating slowly, chewing thoroughly, and appreciating each bite. This practice can improve digestion, help control portion sizes, and reduce the likelihood of overeating. Additionally, taking time to savor your food allows you to make more conscious choices, ensuring that you're nourishing your liver and body properly.

Supplements That Benefit Liver Health

While maintaining a balanced diet and a healthy lifestyle is crucial for liver health, certain supplements can offer additional support. The liver, being one of the body's primary detoxification organs, can benefit from specific nutrients and herbal supplements that aid its ability to detoxify, repair, and regenerate. In this section, we will explore some of the most effective supplements that can support and improve liver function, providing extra protection and enhancing detoxification processes.

Milk Thistle

Milk Thistle (Silybum marianum) is one of the most popular herbal supplements for liver health. It contains a powerful antioxidant compound called **silymarin**, which has been studied extensively for its ability to protect liver cells from damage and promote liver regeneration. Silymarin has shown potential in the treatment of conditions like **non-alcoholic fatty liver disease (NAFLD)**, **alcoholic liver disease**, and **hepatitis**.

Milk thistle works by blocking toxins and free radicals from damaging liver cells, and it has been shown to have anti-inflammatory and liver-protective properties. It also stimulates the production of **glutathione**, one of the body's most powerful antioxidants, which aids the liver in detoxifying harmful substances. Additionally, milk thistle has been found to improve liver function markers, such as **ALT** (alanine transaminase) and **AST** (aspartate transaminase), which are often elevated in individuals with liver disease.

Dandelion Root

Dandelion Root (Taraxacum officinale) has been used for centuries as a natural remedy for liver and digestive health. This herb is rich in antioxidants, vitamins, and minerals that support liver detoxification and bile production. Dandelion root helps the liver by stimulating its natural detoxification processes and encouraging the elimination of toxins and waste products.

Dandelion root also promotes bile flow, which helps in the digestion of fats and the removal of waste from the body. Some studies have indicated that dandelion root may also assist in reducing inflammation and protecting liver cells from oxidative stress, making it a valuable supplement for liver health, especially for those dealing with liver congestion or sluggish bile flow.

Artichoke Extract

Artichoke Extract (Cynara scolymus) is another supplement that has gained popularity due to its liver-supporting benefits. Artichoke is rich in **cynarin**, a compound known to stimulate bile production and improve digestion. This herb is beneficial for individuals suffering from conditions such as **gallbladder issues**, **fatty liver disease**, and **digestive disorders**.

Artichoke extract has been shown to help lower **cholesterol levels**, improve liver enzyme levels, and promote the regeneration of liver cells. Additionally, the antioxidants in artichoke extract help protect the liver from oxidative damage and support the liver's detoxification pathways. Incorporating artichoke extract into your daily routine can support liver function and improve overall digestive health.

Essential Vitamins: Vitamin C, Vitamin E, and B Vitamins

In addition to herbal supplements, specific vitamins are essential for maintaining liver health. Vitamins are crucial for cellular repair, immune function, and the detoxification processes that occur within the liver. Among the many vitamins, **Vitamin C**, **Vitamin E**, and **B Vitamins** are particularly important for supporting liver health.

Vitamin C

Vitamin C (ascorbic acid) is a powerful antioxidant that plays a key role in protecting liver cells from oxidative damage caused by free radicals. The liver, being one of the body's primary detoxifying organs, is constantly exposed to toxins and metabolic waste, making it vulnerable to oxidative stress. Vitamin C helps neutralize free radicals, preventing cellular damage and supporting the liver's ability to repair itself.

Moreover, Vitamin C is essential for the production of **collagen**, which is important for liver tissue repair, especially in individuals suffering from liver cirrhosis or other forms of liver damage. It also plays a role in **boosting the immune system**, helping to prevent infections that can further stress the liver. To support liver health, consume foods rich in Vitamin C, such as **oranges, strawberries, bell peppers**, and **broccoli**. You may also consider taking a Vitamin C supplement, particularly during times of increased oxidative stress.

Vitamin E

Vitamin E is another potent antioxidant that is critical for liver health. It helps protect liver cells from the damaging effects of oxidative stress and inflammation, both of which can contribute to liver disease. Vitamin E has been shown to be particularly beneficial for individuals with **non-alcoholic fatty liver disease (NAFLD)**, where it may help reduce liver fat accumulation and inflammation.

Vitamin E also supports the liver's detoxification pathways and enhances the body's ability to process and eliminate harmful substances. It has been shown to improve liver function in individuals with liver disease, and its antioxidant properties play a crucial role in protecting the liver from long-term damage. Foods rich in Vitamin E include **sunflower seeds**, **almonds**, **spinach**, and **avocados**. Supplements may be considered, but it is important to use them under the guidance of a healthcare professional, as high doses of Vitamin E can cause side effects.

B Vitamins

B Vitamins, particularly **Vitamin B12**, **B6**, and **Folate**, are vital for liver function. These vitamins play a role in the production of enzymes that aid in the metabolism of fats, proteins, and carbohydrates. They also support the liver in its detoxification efforts, making them essential for anyone looking to improve liver health.

Vitamin **B12** is important for maintaining healthy nerve cells and red blood cells, as well as for metabolizing fats and carbohydrates. **Vitamin B6** aids in the breakdown of proteins and supports detoxification, while **Folate** helps with DNA repair and cell regeneration. All three B vitamins play a role in reducing liver inflammation and promoting liver cell repair. Good dietary sources of B vitamins include **meat, fish, eggs**, and **leafy greens**, or you may consider a **B-complex** supplement.

Antioxidants and Liver Protection

Antioxidants are substances that help protect the body from **oxidative stress** caused by free radicals, which can damage cells and lead to inflammation. The liver, in its role as the body's primary detoxifier, is especially vulnerable to oxidative stress. Therefore, consuming antioxidant-rich foods and supplements is crucial for supporting liver health and preventing liver diseases such as cirrhosis, fatty liver disease, and hepatitis.

The Role of Antioxidants in Liver Health

The liver contains specialized enzymes that help neutralize toxins, but these enzymes require antioxidants to work effectively. Antioxidants, such as **Vitamin C**, **Vitamin E**, **selenium**, and **glutathione**, help neutralize free radicals, reduce liver inflammation, and support the liver's detoxification processes. These antioxidants can be found in a variety of foods, including fruits, vegetables, nuts, seeds, and green tea.

For instance, **green tea** is packed with **catechins**, a type of antioxidant that has been shown to improve liver function and reduce liver fat. **Beta-carotene**, found in **carrots** and **sweet potatoes**, is another antioxidant that supports liver health by reducing oxidative damage and promoting liver cell regeneration.

In addition to eating antioxidant-rich foods, you may consider **supplements** such as **milk thistle**, which contains silymarin, an antioxidant that protects liver cells and supports their regeneration. Other supplements, like **curcumin** (found in turmeric), have powerful antioxidant properties that help reduce liver inflammation and oxidative stress, promoting overall liver health.

Liver Detoxification and Antioxidants

The liver plays a major role in detoxification by breaking down toxins and chemicals into safer compounds that can be eliminated from the body. Antioxidants support the liver's detoxification abilities by reducing oxidative stress and enhancing its detoxifying processes. Certain antioxidants, such as **glutathione**, are produced by the liver and are crucial for breaking down harmful substances.

Incorporating antioxidant-rich foods like **berries, green leafy vegetables, garlic, and artichokes** into your diet helps support the liver's detoxification functions. You may also consider taking specific antioxidant supplements to further protect the liver from damage.

Chapter 6: Natural Remedies for Fatty Liver and Inflammation

Herbal and Natural Solutions for Fatty Liver

Fatty liver disease is a common and often silent condition that affects millions of people worldwide. It occurs when excess fat builds up in the liver, a vital organ responsible for processing toxins, producing bile, and storing energy. There are two main types of fatty liver disease: alcoholic and non-alcoholic fatty liver disease (NAFLD). While alcohol consumption is a major risk factor for fatty liver disease, NAFLD is closely linked to obesity, diabetes, poor diet, and a sedentary lifestyle.

Fortunately, nature offers a wide variety of herbal and natural remedies that can help manage and even reverse fatty liver disease. The use of plants for healing has been passed down through generations, and modern research supports their effectiveness in treating liver conditions. When considering natural remedies for fatty liver, it's important to focus on those that reduce inflammation, support liver detoxification, and improve overall liver function.

1. Dandelion Root (Taraxacum officinale)

Dandelion root has been used for centuries in traditional medicine to treat liver conditions. It is known for its ability to stimulate bile production, helping the liver process fat more effectively. Bile is essential for the digestion and absorption of fats, and by enhancing bile flow, dandelion root helps reduce fat accumulation in the liver. Studies have shown that dandelion root also has antioxidant and anti-inflammatory properties, both of which are crucial for reversing fatty liver disease.

2. Milk Thistle (Silybum marianum)

Milk thistle is one of the most researched and well-known herbs for liver health. Its active compound, silymarin, is a powerful antioxidant that protects liver cells from damage caused by free radicals. Silymarin also has anti-inflammatory properties, making it effective in reducing the inflammation commonly seen in fatty liver disease. This herb helps promote liver regeneration by encouraging the growth of new liver cells and improving liver function. Milk thistle has been shown to reduce liver enzyme levels and improve liver health in patients with both alcoholic and non-alcoholic fatty liver disease (NAFLD).

3. Artichoke (Cynara scolymus)

Artichoke has long been valued for its liver-protective effects. It contains cynarin, a compound that stimulates bile production and improves fat digestion. This action reduces the burden on the liver, preventing fat from accumulating. Artichoke also has antioxidant properties, which help protect liver cells from oxidative stress. Regular consumption of artichoke extract has been found to lower liver enzyme levels and improve liver function in patients with fatty liver disease.

4. Turmeric (Curcuma longa)

Turmeric, a spice often used in Indian cuisine, contains an active compound called curcumin, which has powerful anti-inflammatory and antioxidant properties. Curcumin has been shown to reduce liver inflammation and protect liver cells from oxidative damage. It also promotes bile production, helping the liver process fats more efficiently. Regular use of turmeric or curcumin supplements can support liver detoxification, reduce fat accumulation, and improve overall liver health.

5. Ginger (Zingiber officinale)

Ginger is another potent herb with liver-protective properties. It has been shown to reduce liver inflammation and oxidative stress, both of which contribute to the development of fatty liver disease. Ginger contains compounds called gingerols and shogaols, which help protect liver cells from damage and improve fat metabolism. Adding fresh ginger to your diet or taking ginger supplements can be beneficial for those with fatty liver disease.

6. Green Tea (Camellia sinensis)

Green tea is well-known for its antioxidant properties, primarily due to its high content of catechins, particularly epigallocatechin gallate (EGCG). These compounds help protect liver cells from oxidative damage and reduce fat accumulation in the liver. Several studies have shown that drinking green tea regularly can improve liver function and reduce the severity of fatty liver disease. Green tea also supports weight loss, which can further help reduce fat buildup in the liver.

The Power of Turmeric and Curcumin

Turmeric, often referred to as the "golden spice," has been used for centuries in traditional medicine, particularly in Ayurvedic and Chinese healing practices. The active ingredient in turmeric is curcumin, which has been the subject of numerous scientific studies due to its potent anti-inflammatory, antioxidant, and hepatoprotective (liver-protecting) effects. Turmeric and curcumin are now widely used as natural remedies for various health conditions, including fatty liver disease.

How Turmeric Supports Liver Health

The liver is constantly exposed to toxins from food, the environment, and even the medications we take. Over time, this toxic burden can lead to liver damage, inflammation, and fat accumulation. Curcumin, the active compound in turmeric, is a powerful antioxidant that scavenges free radicals—unstable molecules that damage cells and tissues. By neutralizing free radicals, curcumin helps protect the liver from oxidative stress, which is a key factor in the development of fatty liver disease.

In addition to its antioxidant effects, curcumin has strong anti-inflammatory properties. Inflammation is one of the primary mechanisms behind fatty liver disease, and curcumin has been shown to reduce liver inflammation, which helps prevent further liver damage and encourages the healing process. Several studies have demonstrated that curcumin supplementation can lower levels of inflammatory markers in individuals with fatty liver disease, improving liver function and reducing fat buildup.

Turmeric's Role in Reducing Fat Accumulation

Curcumin also has the ability to regulate lipid metabolism, which is crucial for preventing fat accumulation in the liver. By improving fat metabolism and supporting the liver's ability to process and eliminate fats, curcumin helps reduce the fat stored in the liver. This can significantly reduce the risk of developing more severe forms of liver disease, such as cirrhosis or liver fibrosis.

Several studies have shown that curcumin supplementation can reduce liver fat content in individuals with non-alcoholic fatty liver disease (NAFLD). In one clinical trial, participants who took curcumin supplements experienced a significant reduction in liver fat and improved liver enzyme levels. These findings suggest that curcumin may be a valuable addition to a treatment regimen for fatty liver disease.

How to Incorporate Turmeric into Your Diet

The most common way to incorporate turmeric into your diet is through food and beverages. Turmeric can be added to soups, curries, stews, and smoothies. However, curcumin is not easily absorbed by the body on its own. To enhance its absorption, it is often recommended to take turmeric with black pepper, which contains piperine, a compound that enhances curcumin absorption by up to 2000%. Additionally, consuming turmeric with healthy fats, such as olive oil or coconut oil, can further increase absorption.

For those looking for higher doses or therapeutic benefits, curcumin supplements are available in various forms, including capsules, tablets, and powders. It's important to consult with a healthcare provider before starting curcumin supplementation, especially if you are taking other medications.

Milk Thistle: The Most Popular Liver Detoxifier

Milk thistle (Silybum marianum) is one of the most widely used herbs for liver health. The active compound in milk thistle is silymarin, which is a group of flavonoids that possess strong antioxidant and anti-inflammatory properties. Silymarin has been extensively studied for its ability to protect and regenerate liver cells, making it a popular choice for people with liver diseases, including fatty liver.

The Science Behind Milk Thistle and Liver Health

Silymarin acts as a potent antioxidant that helps neutralize harmful free radicals in the liver, preventing oxidative damage to liver cells. Oxidative stress is a major contributor to the development of fatty liver disease and other liver conditions, and by reducing oxidative stress, milk thistle helps protect the liver from further damage.

Silymarin also has anti-inflammatory effects, which help reduce liver inflammation—a common feature of fatty liver disease.

In addition to its antioxidant and anti-inflammatory properties, silymarin has been shown to promote liver cell regeneration. This is particularly important in individuals with fatty liver disease, as the liver's ability to regenerate itself is crucial for healing. By encouraging the growth of new liver cells, silymarin helps repair damaged liver tissue and restore normal liver function.

Milk Thistle for Fatty Liver Disease

Milk thistle has been shown to be effective in reducing liver enzyme levels and improving liver function in individuals with fatty liver disease. Several clinical studies have demonstrated that silymarin supplementation can help reduce liver fat content, lower liver enzyme levels, and improve liver health in people with both alcoholic and non-alcoholic fatty liver disease (NAFLD).

One study published in the *World Journal of Gastroenterology* found that milk thistle supplementation led to significant improvements in liver function and a reduction in liver fat in individuals with NAFLD. Other studies have shown that milk thistle can reduce symptoms associated with liver disease, such as fatigue and bloating, and improve overall quality of life.

How to Use Milk Thistle

Milk thistle is available in various forms, including capsules, tablets, liquid extracts, and teas. The most common dosage used in studies is 140-420 mg of silymarin per day, divided into two or three doses. It's important to consult with a healthcare provider before starting milk thistle supplementation, especially if you have liver disease or are taking other medications.

For those who prefer a more natural approach, milk thistle can be consumed as a tea. However, the concentration of silymarin in tea is much lower compared to supplements, so it may not be as effective for treating liver disease on its own.

How to Reduce Liver Inflammation Naturally

Liver inflammation, also known as **hepatitis**, can be caused by infections, toxins, an unhealthy diet, or autoimmune conditions. When the liver is inflamed, it cannot function properly, leading to fatigue, digestive problems, and even serious liver diseases like cirrhosis or liver failure. Fortunately, there are many natural ways to reduce liver inflammation and restore optimal liver function. Let's explore them in detail.

1. Eliminate Toxins from Your Life

One of the biggest culprits behind liver inflammation is the constant exposure to toxins. These toxins come from processed foods, alcohol, pollution, medications, and even personal care products. The first step to healing your liver is to reduce your toxic load.

a) Avoid Processed Foods

Processed foods contain high amounts of **refined sugars, unhealthy fats, and artificial additives** that burden the liver. Choose fresh, whole foods instead, such as vegetables, fruits, nuts, seeds, and lean proteins.

b) Reduce Alcohol Intake

Alcohol is one of the most damaging substances for the liver. It causes oxidative stress, leads to fat buildup, and triggers inflammation. If you want to heal your liver, it's best to avoid alcohol completely or limit it to **one drink per week**.

c) Switch to Natural Cleaning and Personal Care Products

Many household cleaners, cosmetics, and skincare products contain toxic chemicals that the liver must detoxify. Opt for natural alternatives made from plant-based ingredients to reduce the burden on your liver.

2. Adopt a Liver-Healing Diet

a) Increase Your Intake of Anti-Inflammatory Foods

Certain foods have powerful anti-inflammatory properties that help repair liver cells and reduce swelling. Some of the best foods for liver inflammation include:

- **Leafy Greens:** Spinach, kale, and arugula help neutralize toxins.
- **Cruciferous Vegetables:** Broccoli, Brussels sprouts, and cauliflower enhance liver detoxification.
- **Berries:** Blueberries, raspberries, and blackberries are rich in antioxidants.
- **Fatty Fish:** Salmon and sardines contain omega-3 fatty acids, which combat liver inflammation.

b) Drink Liver-Healing Beverages

What you drink is just as important as what you eat. **Dandelion tea, green tea, lemon water, and beet juice** are fantastic for reducing inflammation and improving liver function.

c) Reduce Sugar and Refined Carbs

Excess sugar leads to **fatty liver disease**, which worsens inflammation. Reduce consumption of white bread, pastries, soda, and processed snacks. Instead, opt for natural sweeteners like honey or dates in moderation.

3. Support Your Gut Health

The liver and gut are deeply connected. A **healthy gut microbiome** can significantly reduce liver inflammation. To improve gut health:

- Eat **fermented foods** like yogurt, kefir, sauerkraut, and kimchi.
- Take **probiotic supplements** to restore good bacteria in the gut.
- Increase **fiber intake** to improve digestion and prevent the buildup of harmful toxins.

4. Stay Hydrated

Drinking **enough water** is essential for liver function. Water helps flush out toxins, reduces stress on the liver, and keeps inflammation under control. Aim for at least **8–10 glasses** of water per day.

5. Get Quality Sleep

Your liver performs most of its detoxification while you sleep. Poor sleep disrupts this process and increases inflammation. Aim for **7–9 hours** of quality sleep every night by:

- Avoiding caffeine in the evening.
- Keeping a regular sleep schedule.
- Reducing screen time before bed.

6. Engage in Gentle Exercise

Moderate exercise **reduces fat buildup in the liver, lowers inflammation, and improves overall liver function**. Low-impact exercises like walking, yoga, swimming, or tai chi are particularly beneficial.

7. Reduce Stress

Chronic stress leads to hormonal imbalances that **worsen liver inflammation**. Practice stress management techniques such as **deep breathing, meditation, or spending time in nature**.

8. Use Natural Supplements for Liver Support

Several natural supplements have been proven to **reduce liver inflammation**:

- **Milk Thistle:** Protects liver cells and reduces oxidative stress.
- **Turmeric:** Contains curcumin, a powerful anti-inflammatory compound.
- **NAC (N-Acetyl Cysteine):** Helps detoxify the liver.
- **Omega-3 Fatty Acids:** Reduces fat buildup and inflammation in the liver.

Reducing liver inflammation naturally requires a **holistic approach**—eliminating toxins, eating anti-inflammatory foods, managing stress, and prioritizing sleep. By following these steps, you can help your liver heal and function at its best.

Supporting Liver Function with Hydration

Hydration is one of the most important and often overlooked factors in maintaining overall health. For the liver, proper hydration supports its detoxifying processes, enhances its efficiency, and reduces the burden of toxins in the body. Let's take a closer look at how hydration specifically supports liver function and why it is crucial for a healthy liver.

The liver is the body's primary organ for detoxification. It filters toxins, waste products, and chemicals from the bloodstream. This role is vital for our survival, yet it can only be effectively carried out when the liver is well-supported by the body's hydration status. If the liver lacks sufficient fluids, its ability to break down and remove toxins diminishes, leading to a backlog of waste products in the body. This situation can cause fatigue, digestive issues, and general malaise, which are common signs of liver stress.

Water: The Liver's Best Friend

Water plays a direct role in liver health by facilitating its detoxification functions. The liver uses water to help break down harmful substances in the body, which are then flushed out through the kidneys and bladder. When you drink adequate amounts of water, you provide your liver with the resources it needs to filter out toxins, waste products, and excess nutrients.

Water also helps maintain the flow of bile, the digestive fluid produced by the liver. Bile is essential for digesting fats and absorbing fat-soluble vitamins (A, D, E, K). Without enough water, bile becomes thick and viscous, making it harder for the liver to secrete it and for the digestive system to utilize it. This can lead to digestive discomfort, sluggishness, and a feeling of heaviness in the body.

How Much Water Does the Liver Need?

The recommended daily water intake varies depending on factors like body size, activity level, and climate. On average, a healthy adult should aim to drink at least 8 cups (64 ounces) of water per day. However, when the liver is under additional stress, such as during detoxification, this amount may need to be increased. Keep in mind that water from food sources (such as fruits and vegetables) and other fluids (like herbal teas) contribute to overall hydration levels as well.

Electrolytes: A Crucial Component for Liver Function

Hydration isn't just about water – electrolytes play a pivotal role in maintaining balance within the body's fluid systems. Electrolytes, including sodium, potassium, magnesium, and calcium, help regulate fluid balance, nerve function, and muscle function. When it comes to liver health, electrolytes help maintain blood pressure and proper blood flow to the liver, ensuring that the organ is receiving the nutrients and oxygen it needs to function optimally.

Signs Your Liver Might Be Dehydrated

It's important to pay attention to signs of dehydration. These can include dry skin, dry mouth, fatigue, dizziness, and dark urine. If you are experiencing any of these symptoms, it's essential to increase your water intake and restore electrolyte balance. You can replenish electrolytes naturally through foods like bananas, avocados, leafy greens, and nuts, or consider electrolyte-enhanced beverages that don't contain added sugars or artificial additives.

The Bottom Line on Hydration for Liver Health

Proper hydration is an essential part of liver health. By drinking sufficient water, replenishing electrolytes, and maintaining a balanced diet, you can help your liver function at its best.

Remember, the liver works tirelessly to detoxify the body, and by supporting it with adequate hydration, you can ensure that it remains efficient in its role, keeping you feeling vibrant and healthy.

The Role of Water and Electrolytes in Liver Health

When discussing hydration, it's important to highlight not just the role of water, but also the critical function of electrolytes. Electrolytes are minerals that conduct electrical impulses in the body, and they play a vital role in various bodily functions, including liver health. Here, we will dive deeper into why both water and electrolytes are indispensable for maintaining liver function and how to balance them for optimal liver health.

Understanding Electrolytes and Their Function in the Body

Electrolytes are essential for maintaining the balance of fluids in the body, ensuring proper nerve and muscle function, regulating the acid-base balance, and supporting hydration. Key electrolytes such as sodium, potassium, calcium, and magnesium influence not only cellular functions but also processes like blood circulation and detoxification, both of which are critical to liver health.

The liver has to filter large amounts of blood each day, extracting toxins and waste products that need to be removed from the body. Electrolytes play a role in regulating the volume and pressure of blood as it flows through the liver. When electrolytes are out of balance, blood flow to the liver can become impaired, and the liver may not be able to process toxins as efficiently.

How Dehydration Affects Liver Function

Dehydration impacts liver health in many ways. When the body becomes dehydrated, the liver loses its ability to perform its detoxifying and metabolic functions efficiently. This can result in a buildup of toxins in the blood, which can damage liver cells over time. Dehydration can also lead to bile becoming more concentrated and less able to flow freely, which can lead to digestive issues, constipation, and even gallstones.

Hydrated cells are more effective at eliminating toxins, and this is crucial for the liver. Electrolyte imbalance caused by dehydration can also compromise liver detox pathways, which is why maintaining hydration with the right electrolytes is essential for keeping the liver in top working order.

The Importance of Sodium and Potassium for Liver Health

Sodium and potassium are two of the most important electrolytes for liver function. Sodium is responsible for maintaining fluid balance in the body, while potassium helps regulate the balance of fluids within cells, tissues, and organs. Both sodium and potassium play a role in controlling blood pressure, which affects the delivery of oxygen and nutrients to the liver.

If either of these electrolytes is too low or too high, it can impair liver function. For example, low potassium levels (hypokalemia) can lead to muscle weakness, fatigue, and constipation. Conversely, excess sodium (hypernatremia) can result in fluid retention, which places additional strain on the liver's ability to filter toxins.

Magnesium: The Unsung Hero of Liver Detoxification

Magnesium is another key electrolyte that supports liver function. This mineral is involved in over 300 enzymatic reactions in the body, many of which are related to liver detoxification. Magnesium plays a role in breaking down toxins and helps the liver process fat, protein, and carbohydrates. A deficiency in magnesium can cause liver cells to become less efficient at detoxifying, which can lead to fatty liver disease and other metabolic disorders.

Maintaining Electrolyte Balance for Liver Health

Maintaining a balanced intake of electrolytes is essential for optimal liver health. Hydration with electrolytes can be supported through the consumption of water, foods, and beverages rich in minerals. Natural sources of electrolytes include fruits and vegetables like bananas, sweet potatoes, spinach, and oranges. Coconut water is also a popular natural electrolyte drink that can help replenish both fluids and electrolytes in the body.

If you're looking to add more hydration support, electrolyte tablets or powders can be added to your water, but it's important to choose ones that don't contain added sugars or artificial ingredients.

The Role of Hydration in Preventing Liver Disease

Proper hydration combined with electrolyte balance can be preventive in nature. When the liver is well-hydrated, its ability to detoxify and filter toxins is greatly improved. This can prevent conditions like fatty liver disease, hepatitis, cirrhosis, and even liver cancer. Hydration aids in the maintenance of liver enzymes, allowing for efficient metabolic processes and reducing the buildup of harmful substances in the body.

Herbal Teas and Infusions for Liver Detox

Herbal teas and infusions have long been used in traditional medicine as natural remedies for various health issues, including liver detoxification. While the liver is naturally equipped to detoxify itself, certain herbs can enhance the process, providing additional support.

Let's take a look at the most effective herbs and teas known for their liver detox properties.

Milk Thistle: The Gold Standard for Liver Health

Milk thistle is one of the most well-known herbs for liver health. It contains an active compound called silymarin, which has been shown to have potent antioxidant and anti-inflammatory properties. Silymarin helps protect liver cells from damage caused by toxins, alcohol, and other harmful substances. It also promotes the regeneration of liver cells, making it an excellent herb for liver detox and repair.

Milk thistle can be consumed as a tea, extract, or supplement. Drinking milk thistle tea regularly can help to support liver function and protect the liver from toxins, reducing the risk of conditions like fatty liver disease and cirrhosis.

Dandelion Root: A Natural Liver Cleanser

Dandelion root is another herb known for its detoxifying effects. It is particularly effective in promoting bile production, which is crucial for digestion and the elimination of toxins from the liver. Dandelion root tea acts as a mild diuretic, helping the body flush out excess water and toxins.

In addition to supporting liver detoxification, dandelion root also has anti-inflammatory properties, making it useful for reducing liver inflammation. Drinking dandelion root tea regularly can help the liver filter out toxins more efficiently and keep the digestive system running smoothly.

Turmeric: The Anti-Inflammatory Super Herb

Turmeric contains curcumin, a compound with powerful anti-inflammatory and antioxidant properties. Curcumin has been found to help reduce liver inflammation and promote detoxification by enhancing bile production. Turmeric tea, made with fresh or powdered turmeric root, can support liver function, improve digestion, and reduce oxidative stress in the liver.

Turmeric also helps reduce fat accumulation in the liver, making it a useful herb for preventing and managing fatty liver disease.

Other Herbal Teas for Liver Detox

Several other herbal teas can support liver detoxification, including:

- **Ginger Tea**: Known for its anti-inflammatory properties, ginger supports the digestive system and helps stimulate bile production in the liver.
- **Peppermint Tea**: Peppermint can aid digestion and reduce liver congestion by promoting bile flow.
- **Lemon Balm Tea**: This herb has calming properties and can help reduce liver stress, supporting liver detoxification.

Conclusion on Herbal Teas for Liver Detox

Incorporating herbal teas and infusions into your daily routine can be an effective way to support liver health. Herbs like milk thistle, dandelion root, and turmeric are especially beneficial for detoxifying the liver, reducing inflammation, and promoting bile production.

Benefits of Bone Broth and Fresh Juices

Bone broth and fresh juices are excellent ways to support liver health through natural, nutrient-dense liquids that promote detoxification and healing.

Bone Broth: A Nutrient Powerhouse for the Liver

Bone broth is made by simmering bones and connective tissues for an extended period, allowing the minerals, collagen, and amino acids to be extracted into the liquid. These nutrients can support liver health by providing essential building blocks for tissue repair and reducing inflammation.

Bone broth contains glycine, an amino acid that has been shown to have protective effects on the liver. Glycine helps reduce liver inflammation and protects liver cells from oxidative stress. It also supports the liver's detoxification processes, promoting the elimination of harmful toxins from the body.

Fresh Juices: A Liver Detox in a Glass

Fresh juices made from fruits and vegetables are rich in antioxidants, vitamins, and minerals that can aid liver detoxification. Juices made from ingredients like beets, carrots, and apples are particularly beneficial for the liver, as they support detox pathways and promote bile flow.

Beet juice is especially well-known for its liver-cleansing properties. Beets are high in betalains, compounds that support liver detoxification and protect the liver from damage. Carrot juice is rich in beta-carotene, which helps protect liver cells from oxidative damage and promotes liver regeneration.

Chapter 7: Liver-Friendly Exercise and Lifestyle Habits

The liver is often regarded as the body's detoxification powerhouse. It works tirelessly to filter out toxins, process nutrients, and metabolize substances vital for our survival. However, just like any other organ, it requires care and attention. Our modern-day lifestyle, full of poor diet choices, lack of movement, and environmental toxins, can put undue stress on the liver. Thankfully, lifestyle adjustments, especially incorporating exercise, can work wonders in supporting liver health.

Exercise isn't just about maintaining a healthy weight—it's also about improving the liver's ability to perform its detoxifying and metabolic functions. The right kind of exercise can reduce liver fat, improve liver enzyme levels, and help prevent or manage liver diseases like fatty liver disease and cirrhosis. When combined with healthy habits, regular exercise is one of the most powerful tools we have in maintaining liver health.

The Best Types of Exercise for Liver Health

Before we dive into specific types of exercises, let's take a moment to understand how exercise benefits the liver.

When we engage in physical activity, we increase blood flow, which helps the liver function more efficiently. Exercise also improves insulin sensitivity, which is critical for regulating blood sugar and preventing fatty liver disease, a common ailment related to poor lifestyle habits. By reducing fat deposits in the liver, exercise helps alleviate the burden on this vital organ.

The best types of exercise for liver health generally include aerobic activities, strength training, and stretching exercises. Let's look at each one more closely.

Aerobic Exercise: Walking, Running, Swimming

Aerobic exercise, also known as cardio, involves activities that increase your heart rate and improve cardiovascular endurance. These exercises work wonders for liver health by helping reduce fatty deposits in the liver and improving overall liver function.

Walking: One of the simplest and most accessible forms of aerobic exercise is walking. It requires no special equipment or facilities, and it's easy to incorporate into your daily routine. Whether you're strolling around the block, walking at a brisk pace, or taking a hike in the park, walking can help burn calories, reduce liver fat, and lower stress levels.

For liver health, aim for at least 30 minutes of brisk walking five times a week. Regular walking has been shown to improve liver enzyme levels, reduce the risk of developing non-alcoholic fatty liver disease (NAFLD), and lower your chances of other chronic conditions such as diabetes and high blood pressure.

Running: For those who are a bit more athletic or prefer higher intensity activities, running is an excellent form of exercise. Running elevates your heart rate, helping to burn fat and calories more efficiently than walking. Studies have shown that regular running significantly reduces the amount of fat in the liver, making it a vital exercise for those looking to manage or prevent fatty liver disease.

Running also helps improve insulin sensitivity, which is essential for liver health, as insulin resistance is a major risk factor for NAFLD and other metabolic conditions. If you're new to running, start with shorter distances and gradually increase your stamina over time.

Swimming: Swimming is a low-impact aerobic exercise that is particularly beneficial for people with joint pain or those who are overweight. The buoyancy of the water reduces strain on the joints while still providing an effective cardiovascular workout. Swimming helps burn fat and improve overall cardiovascular health, which in turn supports liver function.

Like other aerobic exercises, swimming helps regulate blood sugar levels, reduce fat in the liver, and improve liver enzyme activity. It's an excellent choice for anyone looking to stay fit while also supporting liver health.

Strength Training and Its Effects on Liver Fat

Strength training, also known as resistance training, involves exercises where muscles work against an external resistance. This resistance can come from free weights, machines, or even bodyweight exercises such as push-ups and squats. Strength training is often associated with building muscle mass and improving bone density, but its benefits extend to liver health as well.

How Strength Training Supports Liver Health:
Strength training can help reduce liver fat in a unique way. Unlike aerobic exercises, which primarily burn fat during the activity, strength training helps increase muscle mass over time. Muscles are metabolically active tissues, meaning they burn more calories even when you're not exercising. This increased calorie burn can lead to weight loss and reduced fat accumulation in the liver, ultimately benefiting liver function.

Studies have shown that strength training improves insulin sensitivity, a critical factor in liver health. People who engage in regular strength training see a reduction in visceral fat (fat that accumulates around the liver) and a decrease in liver enzymes associated with liver damage.

Best Strength Training Exercises for Liver Health:

1. **Squats and Lunges:** These exercises target large muscle groups in the lower body and help build muscle mass. Using weights increases the intensity, leading to more significant muscle growth and fat burning.

2. **Push-ups and Pull-ups:** These exercises engage the upper body muscles, such as the chest, arms, and back. They can be done anywhere without equipment, making them convenient for home workouts.

3. **Deadlifts and Rows:** These compound movements engage multiple muscle groups, including the legs, back, and core. They are excellent for building overall strength and improving metabolism.

To reap the benefits of strength training for liver health, aim to perform full-body workouts at least two to three times a week. Start with lighter weights and increase the intensity as your muscles become accustomed to the training.

Yoga and Stretching for Detoxification

Yoga and stretching exercises are often overlooked in discussions about liver health, but they play an essential role in promoting detoxification, reducing stress, and improving overall wellness.

Yoga is a holistic practice that combines physical postures, breathing exercises, and meditation, all of which benefit the liver.

How Yoga Benefits Liver Health:
Certain yoga poses stimulate the liver directly, promoting the flow of blood and energy to this vital organ. Additionally, the deep breathing exercises practiced in yoga help activate the diaphragm and stimulate the body's detoxification processes. Yoga also has a calming effect on the nervous system, which helps reduce stress—a major contributor to liver problems like fatty liver disease and cirrhosis.

Specific Yoga Poses for Liver Health:

1. **The Seated Twist (Ardha Matsyendrasana):** This twisting pose helps massage the abdominal organs, including the liver, and promotes detoxification by stimulating the digestive system.

2. **Downward Dog (Adho Mukha Svanasana):** This inverted pose increases blood flow to the head and liver, helping to rejuvenate the body and reduce fat accumulation in the liver.

3. **Bridge Pose (Setu Bandhasana):** This pose gently stimulates the liver and kidneys while also stretching the spine and hips, helping to improve posture and reduce tension in the body.

Stretching and Detoxification:
Stretching exercises, when done regularly, help improve flexibility, reduce muscle tension, and increase blood flow. Specific stretches can target the liver area, improving its function by promoting better

circulation. Gentle stretches like side bends and hip openers can help release trapped energy and toxins, contributing to overall liver health.

Integrating Exercise into Your Daily Routine

Incorporating liver-friendly exercise into your daily life doesn't have to be complicated. The key is consistency. Whether you prefer brisk walking, intense running, strength training, or a calming yoga session, make exercise a non-negotiable part of your routine. Here are a few tips to help you get started:

1. **Start Slow:** If you're new to exercise, begin with 10-15 minutes of light activity and gradually build up to longer sessions. Over time, your body will adapt, and you'll notice improvements in your fitness levels and overall health.

2. **Make It Enjoyable:** Choose activities that you enjoy so you're more likely to stick with them. Whether it's swimming, hiking, or dancing, find something that brings you joy.

3. **Consistency Is Key:** Aim for at least 150 minutes of moderate-intensity aerobic exercise each week, along with strength training sessions twice a week. Consistency is crucial for long-term liver health.

4. **Listen to Your Body:** If you experience pain or discomfort while exercising, stop and seek medical advice. The goal is to promote health, not cause injury.

Regular exercise is an incredibly effective way to support liver health, reduce fat deposits, improve liver function, and prevent liver diseases. Whether it's aerobic exercise, strength training, or yoga, each type of exercise offers unique benefits for the liver. The combination of these exercises, along with a healthy diet and lifestyle, can significantly enhance the liver's ability to detoxify, metabolize, and regenerate. By making these practices part of your routine, you are giving your liver the care it deserves and ensuring a healthier, more vibrant life.

Incorporating Movement into Daily Life

As a seasoned medical professional, one of the most common pieces of advice I give to my patients is the importance of incorporating movement into daily life. Movement isn't just about going to the gym or following a strict exercise routine; it's about finding opportunities to move throughout the day, no matter how busy or constrained by health conditions you might feel.

In my many years of experience, I've seen firsthand how a sedentary lifestyle can silently cause a host of health problems—from weight gain to heart disease, to liver issues and even mental health struggles like anxiety and depression. The human body is designed for movement. Our muscles, joints, and even our internal organs, like the liver and heart, all function better when we engage in regular movement. But how can we incorporate this into our everyday lives, especially when our schedules seem overwhelmingly full?

1. Start Small and Build Gradually

If you are not used to being active, the first step is to start small. The key here is consistency. You do not need to spend hours in a gym to experience the benefits of movement. Simply walking more, stretching in the morning, or even doing basic house chores can have profound benefits. A simple practice to get started could be walking around your home or office during phone calls. This small step can already make a significant difference in how your body feels.

I always recommend setting realistic goals. For example, try walking for 10 minutes after meals or take the stairs instead of the elevator. Over time, these small adjustments accumulate into more meaningful physical activity.

2. Take Advantage of Downtime

We all have moments in our day where we are waiting—waiting in line, waiting for a meeting to start, or waiting for the kettle to boil. These are perfect opportunities to incorporate movement. While waiting, consider doing some light stretches or walking around the house. If you're at work, try to take a quick walk to get a drink of water or stand up and stretch every 30 minutes.

Many people overlook the benefits of these small movements, but they can add up over the course of the day. If you can't find time to exercise, don't stress—just move more during the moments you can.

3. Incorporate Movement into Family Time

If you're a parent or caregiver, this one's for you. It's easy to think that you have no time for movement when you're taking care of children or other family members. However, I always tell my patients to turn family time into active time. Play catch with your kids, go for family walks, or even take a trip to the park. These simple activities don't just provide you with quality time together but also with the necessary movement to keep your body healthy.

In fact, many studies have shown that engaging in physical activity with your loved ones increases not only your bond but also the likelihood that the habit will stick. When you make physical activity a part of your daily interactions, it doesn't feel like a chore.

4. Stand More, Sit Less

One of the most detrimental effects of modern living is the sheer amount of time we spend sitting. Whether it's in front of a computer, watching TV, or driving, prolonged sitting can lead to a variety of health problems, including obesity, cardiovascular disease, and poor posture.

It's important to take breaks. Even if you are working long hours at a desk, standing up every 30 minutes or so can make a big difference. You can also try using a standing desk or sitting on a stability ball for a change. These simple modifications help improve posture and increase your overall movement throughout the day.

5. Movement Doesn't Have to Be Intense

Not all movement needs to be high-intensity. If you're recovering from an injury or simply don't have the energy for a strenuous workout, low-impact activities such as swimming, walking, or even gentle yoga can still help keep your body strong and healthy. As we age, it's essential to focus on low-impact activities that reduce strain on joints and muscles.

I've seen many older patients who feel they're "too old" to exercise, but the truth is, gentle movement is even more important as we age. It's never too late to start, and you can benefit from movement no matter your age or physical condition.

How to Stay Active Even with a Busy Schedule

In today's fast-paced world, it often feels like there simply isn't enough time in the day to exercise. Between work, family, and personal commitments, it can be easy to let movement fall to the wayside. However, staying active is crucial for maintaining long-term health, and even a busy schedule doesn't have to get in the way of this essential part of life.

Over the years, I have worked with many patients who believe that they must dedicate hours each week to fitness, but that's simply not the case. The key is to optimize your time and stay consistent. Here are some tips for staying active even when your schedule is packed:

1. Prioritize Movement as Part of Your Daily Routine

The first step is making a conscious decision to prioritize movement. Consider it just as important as eating or sleeping. It's about making movement a part of your day, no matter what else you have going on. For instance, I encourage patients to build small exercises into their morning or evening routines. It could be something as simple as stretching or doing light cardio for 5 minutes before bed.

Incorporate stretches or squats during your morning routine to get the blood flowing. It may seem small, but these mini work-outs add up over the course of a week.

2. Wake Up Earlier

Many people's excuses for not exercising are based on lack of time, but what if you woke up 20 to 30 minutes earlier to prioritize your health? While it may seem hard at first, waking up a bit earlier can help create a new habit. Whether you use this time for a quick workout, yoga, or a brisk walk, the benefits of early-morning movement are profound. Not only does it energize you for the day, but it also sets a positive tone for your entire schedule.

3. Combine Socializing with Activity

Who says you can't have both fun and fitness at the same time? When you're busy, it's easy to let socializing fall off the agenda. But instead of meeting friends for a sedentary meal or a movie, why not meet for a walk, a bike ride, or even a fitness class? These activities not only help you stay active but also serve as a great way to catch up with friends or family. Consider activities like hiking, walking around the park, or even dancing.

4. Break It Into Smaller Segments

You don't have to commit to a 30-minute workout session all at once. You can break it down into smaller segments throughout the day. For example, take a 10-minute walk during lunch, do some stretches in the morning, or use your break time at work for a few minutes of bodyweight exercises.

Breaking up physical activity into smaller parts has been shown to be just as effective as doing a longer session. This method can be particularly helpful for people with demanding schedules.

5. Use Technology to Stay Accountable

There are now many apps and fitness trackers designed to help you stay on track with your movement goals. These tools are fantastic for those with busy schedules because they can remind you to move, log your steps, and track your progress. Whether it's a simple pedometer on your phone or a full fitness tracker, these tools can provide the extra push you need to stay consistent.

Using Exercise to Fight Fatigue and Stress

As an experienced doctor, I've long known the profound effects that exercise can have on both physical and mental health. One of the most notable benefits of regular physical activity is its ability to combat fatigue and reduce stress. For many of my patients who experience both, I always recommend adding exercise to their daily routine.

Fatigue is often the result of both physical and mental exertion, and in today's world, stress is a constant companion for many. But exercise is one of the best ways to alleviate both. Here's why:

1. Exercise Boosts Energy Levels

It may sound counterintuitive, but regular physical activity is one of the best ways to fight fatigue. Although you may feel tired before exercising, the truth is that exercise increases your energy levels in the long run. The more you move, the more blood and oxygen your body pumps to your muscles, which in turn helps to generate energy.

When you engage in cardiovascular exercises like walking, cycling, or swimming, your heart and lungs become more efficient at delivering oxygen to your body. Over time, this improves your stamina and reduces overall fatigue.

2. Exercise Stimulates the Release of Endorphins

Endorphins are the body's natural mood boosters. When you exercise, especially during high-intensity activities like running or lifting weights, your body releases these chemicals. These endorphins not only help reduce pain but also give you an emotional lift. This can help reduce the effects of stress and promote an overall feeling of well-being.

For patients experiencing chronic stress or anxiety, I often recommend regular physical activity because of its mental health benefits. The act of moving your body can help take your mind off worries, providing a mental break and helping to regulate your emotions.

3. Exercise Reduces Cortisol Levels

Cortisol is often called the "stress hormone." When you experience stress, your body releases cortisol, which can increase feelings of fatigue, anxiety, and tension. Regular exercise helps reduce these cortisol levels, making it a great way to fight stress and fatigue simultaneously.

By balancing cortisol with the calming effects of endorphins, exercise helps maintain a healthy stress response. This is particularly important in today's fast-paced world, where stress is almost constant.

4. Exercise Improves Sleep Quality

Exercise, especially aerobic exercises, can help improve sleep quality. This is especially important for individuals suffering from fatigue, as good sleep is essential for rest and recovery. Regular physical activity helps regulate your sleep-wake cycle, leading to deeper, more restorative sleep, which in turn gives you more energy during the day.

However, it's important not to exercise too close to bedtime, as intense physical activity can sometimes make it harder to fall asleep.

5. Exercise as a Stress Outlet

Finally, exercise serves as an effective outlet for stress. When you're feeling overwhelmed or anxious, physical activity provides a healthy way to release pent-up emotions. Whether you choose to go for a jog, engage in yoga, or simply take a brisk walk, exercise allows you to channel stress and tension into something productive.

Even a small change in your daily habits can have profound effects on your well-being. I encourage you to make movement a priority in your life—you'll soon discover the immense rewards it can bring.

The Role of Rest and Sleep in Liver Function

Sleep is a vital, often overlooked, part of maintaining good liver health. While many focus on diet and exercise when it comes to liver care, rest is just as important. Think of sleep as the body's natural maintenance period. During rest, our organs—including the liver—go into "repair mode," and the liver is no exception.

The Liver's Functions During Sleep

To understand the role of sleep in liver function, it's important to recognize what the liver does while we're awake and during sleep. The liver is a key player in detoxification, processing nutrients, regulating metabolism, storing energy, and producing important substances like bile. It is essentially the body's detox center. But like any other organ, the liver needs time to recharge, repair, and renew its resources, and sleep provides this opportunity.

When we sleep, our body goes into a more relaxed state, which allows organs to work more efficiently. During deep sleep, the liver works on detoxifying the body, breaking down fats, proteins, and sugars more effectively. Without adequate rest, these processes can become sluggish or inefficient, putting extra stress on the liver and affecting its ability to perform vital functions.

Sleep and Liver Regeneration

Sleep has a direct link to liver regeneration. The body uses sleep to clear out toxins and cellular waste. The liver, like other organs, undergoes a process of regeneration while we rest. This is crucial because liver cells, when overworked, can become damaged or even die, leading to liver diseases such as cirrhosis or fatty liver disease. Proper rest ensures that these cells have time to recover and repair. Without sleep, this process is impaired, increasing the risk of long-term liver damage.

Sleep and Detoxification

The liver's detoxification processes are also enhanced during sleep. At night, the body's natural detox systems kick into high gear, with the liver acting as the primary filter for toxins. When we're awake, the liver is busy handling the day's nutrients, so the overnight rest period is essential for it to focus on filtering out harmful substances.

Sleep also plays a role in controlling inflammation. Inflammation can negatively affect the liver by increasing the risk of fatty liver disease and other liver-related conditions. Chronic poor sleep or inadequate sleep may lead to an increase in the body's overall inflammation, which can, in turn, stress the liver.

The Impact of Sleep Cycles on Liver Function

Not all sleep is equal when it comes to liver function. Sleep consists of several cycles, including light sleep, deep sleep, and REM (Rapid Eye Movement) sleep. The liver benefits most from the deeper stages of sleep—specifically, deep sleep and the first few hours of

REM sleep. During deep sleep, the body engages in its most profound repair processes, including liver detoxification and cell regeneration.

If your sleep is disrupted, it interferes with these processes. Inconsistent sleep patterns or poor sleep quality can reduce the efficiency of liver regeneration, leaving the liver vulnerable to damage over time.

How Poor Sleep Affects the Liver

Chronic sleep disturbances or inadequate sleep can have a profound negative effect on liver health. These effects are more subtle at first but can accumulate over time, potentially leading to severe liver damage.

Increased Risk of Fatty Liver Disease

One of the primary conditions linked to poor sleep is Non-Alcoholic Fatty Liver Disease (NAFLD). This condition occurs when fat accumulates in liver cells without significant alcohol consumption. Several studies have shown that poor sleep, particularly a lack of deep sleep, is closely associated with an increased risk of developing fatty liver disease. The liver is unable to break down and process fat properly during sleep deprivation, leading to the storage of fat in liver cells.

Inflammation and Liver Damage

Chronic poor sleep can also result in increased inflammation in the body, which, over time, places additional stress on the liver. Inflammation is a key factor in liver diseases like cirrhosis and hepatitis. When the body is deprived of sleep, the immune system becomes more activated, leading to heightened levels of inflammatory cytokines, which can negatively affect liver tissue and worsen pre-existing liver conditions.

Disrupted Detoxification

During inadequate sleep, the body's natural detox processes become less efficient. The liver has less time to carry out its detoxification duties, and as a result, harmful toxins and waste products accumulate in the bloodstream. This can lead to an increase in overall toxicity in the body, further burdening the liver. Over time, this can lead to liver damage and potentially result in the development of serious liver diseases.

Metabolic Disruptions and Liver Stress

Poor sleep is also a significant contributor to metabolic disorders such as insulin resistance, which is closely linked to liver function. Insulin resistance can lead to a condition called steatosis, which is the buildup of fat in the liver. This disrupts normal liver function and can progress to more serious conditions like cirrhosis or even liver cancer if left unaddressed.

Moreover, sleep disturbances affect the balance of hormones that regulate appetite and metabolism. Lack of sleep has been shown to increase hunger and cravings, particularly for high-fat and high-sugar foods, which puts additional stress on the liver.

Liver Enzyme Imbalance

Disrupted sleep patterns can lead to an imbalance in liver enzymes. Liver enzymes such as ALT (Alanine Aminotransferase) and AST (Aspartate Aminotransferase) are important markers of liver function. Poor sleep may cause elevated levels of these enzymes, which are often indicators of liver inflammation or damage. Over time, high levels of these enzymes can signal liver dysfunction and the need for medical attention.

Tips for Improving Sleep Quality

Given the importance of sleep for liver health, it's crucial to adopt strategies that can improve the quality of your sleep. Here are some practical tips for better sleep that can support liver function:

1. Establish a Regular Sleep Schedule

Consistency is key when it comes to sleep. Going to bed and waking up at the same time every day helps regulate the body's internal clock. A regular sleep schedule ensures that your body goes through all the necessary sleep cycles, including the deep, restorative stages that benefit liver function.

2. Create a Sleep-Friendly Environment

Your bedroom should be a sanctuary for rest. Keep your sleeping area cool, dark, and quiet. Exposure to light at night, especially blue light from electronic devices, can interfere with the body's production of melatonin, a hormone that helps regulate sleep. Consider using blackout curtains, and eliminate electronic devices from your bedroom to promote deeper sleep.

3. Limit Caffeine and Alcohol Consumption

Caffeine and alcohol can both disrupt sleep patterns. Caffeine is a stimulant, and drinking it in the afternoon or evening can interfere with your ability to fall asleep. Alcohol, while it may make you feel drowsy, can disrupt the quality of your sleep by preventing you from entering the deeper stages of restorative sleep. Limiting consumption of both can help improve sleep quality.

4. Engage in Regular Exercise

Exercise is a great way to promote better sleep, but timing matters. Engaging in physical activity earlier in the day can help regulate sleep patterns and improve overall sleep quality. Avoid vigorous exercise close to bedtime, as it can have the opposite effect and make it harder to fall asleep.

5. Manage Stress Levels

Chronic stress can negatively impact sleep quality and, by extension, liver function. Practice relaxation techniques such as deep breathing, meditation, or yoga before bedtime to calm your mind and prepare your body for restful sleep.

6. Focus on Sleep Hygiene

Good sleep hygiene involves habits that promote healthy sleep. Avoid large meals right before bed, as they can cause discomfort and indigestion. Also, limit naps during the day, as they can make it harder to fall asleep at night. Additionally, make sure your mattress and pillows are comfortable to support a restful night.

The Importance of Recovery and Self-Care

Liver health, just like overall health, requires consistent attention and care. Recovery is not just about physical rest, but also about mental and emotional well-being. A holistic approach to recovery that includes good sleep, stress management, healthy eating, and exercise is key to maintaining long-term liver health.

Recovery Time for the Liver

The liver has an incredible ability to regenerate, but it requires time and proper care to do so. Consistently sleeping well, managing stress, eating a balanced diet, and staying hydrated will provide the liver with the necessary conditions to recover effectively. If any of these elements are lacking, the liver may become overburdened and unable to repair itself properly.

Self-Care Strategies

Self-care is about taking the time to prioritize your well-being. For liver health, this means adopting a lifestyle that promotes liver function and includes regular exercise, a balanced diet, and plenty of rest. Regular health check-ups are also important for monitoring liver function, especially if you have a history of liver disease or other risk factors.

Mind-Body Connection

Finally, the mind-body connection is crucial for overall health. Mental stress, if left unchecked, can take a toll on your physical health, including liver function. Incorporating mindfulness practices, such as meditation or journaling, can help reduce mental stress, which ultimately benefits the liver.

By maintaining a healthy lifestyle, improving sleep quality, and practicing regular self-care, you can support your liver and overall well-being for years to come.

Chapter 8: Managing Stress and Emotional Health for Liver Healing

The Impact of Chronic Stress on Liver Function

In the pursuit of maintaining liver health, many often overlook the powerful impact that stress has on this essential organ. The liver, which plays a crucial role in detoxifying the body, processing nutrients, and managing metabolic functions, is intimately connected to the body's emotional and psychological state.

Chronic stress, often a product of our fast-paced modern life, can deeply affect the liver's ability to perform its necessary functions. To fully understand this, we need to explore how stress works within the body, how the liver reacts to stress, and why managing emotional health is as important as diet and exercise when it comes to healing the liver.

When you experience stress, your body reacts by releasing hormones like adrenaline and cortisol, commonly referred to as "stress hormones." These hormones prepare the body for what's often termed the "fight or flight" response. This acute stress response is essential for handling short-term threats or dangers but becomes detrimental when it becomes chronic.

Prolonged or chronic stress, on the other hand, leads to an overproduction of these hormones. With constant elevation of cortisol, the liver can become overworked. Normally, the liver acts as a filtration system, detoxifying the blood, removing toxins, and balancing various bodily functions. However, in times of chronic stress, the liver's functions are compromised, leading to liver dysfunction or the development of conditions such as fatty liver disease, cirrhosis, or even liver failure if left untreated.

One of the key ways chronic stress impacts the liver is by increasing the body's overall inflammatory response. Inflammatory markers are higher during periods of stress, which can put additional strain on the liver. The liver, responsible for filtering out harmful substances, is constantly under pressure to manage an inflamed state, leaving it vulnerable to damage over time.

Moreover, chronic stress affects the immune system, making the liver less capable of defending itself against infections or damage. The immune system often mistakenly attacks the liver in a phenomenon known as autoimmune hepatitis, where the body's defenses target liver cells.

How Stress Hampers Liver Detoxification

The liver's primary role is to detoxify the body by processing and eliminating harmful substances, such as alcohol, drugs, environmental toxins, and metabolic waste products. It also converts nutrients into forms that the body can use, processes proteins, and stores energy. Stress, however, can significantly impair this critical detoxification process.

When you're under stress, the body's hormonal balance becomes disrupted, and cortisol levels remain elevated. The presence of high levels of cortisol can directly affect liver enzymes, which are responsible for breaking down toxins in the liver. One of the liver's detox pathways, called the cytochrome P450 system, is particularly sensitive to stress. This system is involved in metabolizing drugs and other harmful substances. When the stress response is prolonged, the system becomes less efficient, slowing down the liver's ability to process and eliminate toxins from the body.

A sluggish detoxification system allows harmful substances to accumulate in the body, placing an additional burden on the liver and increasing the risk of developing liver diseases. Furthermore, high cortisol levels can alter the liver's ability to store glycogen, leading to energy imbalances and further taxing the liver's functionality.

Another issue caused by chronic stress is the negative impact it has on the gut. Stress often leads to digestive problems like constipation, bloating, or diarrhea, which, in turn, affect nutrient absorption. Poor digestion contributes to toxin buildup in the body and places an even greater strain on the liver. When the digestive system is not functioning optimally, the liver must work overtime to filter out the byproducts of incomplete digestion.

Stress and the Gut-Liver Connection

It is essential to understand the direct connection between stress, the gut, and liver health. The relationship between the gut and liver is a complex one, often referred to as the "gut-liver axis." This axis is a two-way communication network where signals from the gut affect the liver, and vice versa. The health of the gut, including the balance of beneficial bacteria in the digestive system, is a critical factor in maintaining liver function.

When stress is present, it disrupts the balance of the gut microbiota, leading to an increase in harmful bacteria and a decrease in beneficial microbes. This imbalance can cause inflammation in the gut, and these inflammatory signals are transmitted to the liver via the portal vein, a blood vessel that directly connects the gut to the liver. The liver, in turn, responds to this inflammation by releasing immune cells, which further exacerbate liver damage.

Moreover, chronic stress can lead to what is known as "leaky gut," where the lining of the intestines becomes compromised. This allows toxins, bacteria, and other harmful substances to enter the bloodstream. The liver, which is tasked with filtering out these toxins, becomes overwhelmed and less effective in performing its detoxifying duties. The resulting toxic buildup can lead to liver inflammation, fibrosis, and other serious liver conditions.

The stress-induced gut dysfunction also affects digestion, leading to the improper breakdown and absorption of nutrients. This causes malabsorption and nutritional deficiencies, which further burden the liver. Without essential vitamins and minerals, the liver's ability to detoxify and repair itself diminishes, contributing to a vicious cycle of liver deterioration.

Practical Tips for Managing Stress and Supporting Liver Healing

Now that we've established how stress can directly impact liver health, let's explore ways to manage stress effectively and support liver healing:

1. Practice Mindfulness and Meditation

Mindfulness practices, including meditation, yoga, and deep breathing exercises, are powerful tools for reducing stress and supporting liver health. Meditation, for instance, activates the parasympathetic nervous system, often referred to as the "rest and digest" system. This helps to reduce cortisol levels, calm the mind, and allow the liver to function optimally.

A regular mindfulness practice can also help break the cycle of negative thoughts and anxiety that often accompany chronic stress. Simply spending 10–15 minutes each day focusing on your breath and allowing your thoughts to settle can create a profound impact on both your emotional and liver health.

2. Improve Sleep Quality

Lack of sleep or poor-quality sleep can exacerbate stress and lead to increased cortisol production. Ensuring adequate rest is essential for both stress management and liver recovery. Aim for 7-9 hours of sleep per night, and establish a calming nighttime routine to signal your body that it's time to unwind. Limiting screen time before bed, reducing caffeine intake, and creating a peaceful sleep environment can all improve sleep quality.

3. Regular Physical Activity

Exercise is one of the best ways to reduce stress and improve liver function. Regular physical activity helps to lower cortisol levels, promote the release of endorphins (the body's natural mood enhancers), and improve blood circulation, including to the liver. Exercise also supports healthy weight management, reducing the risk of non-alcoholic fatty liver disease (NAFLD), which is often exacerbated by stress and poor lifestyle choices.

Incorporate activities like walking, swimming, cycling, or strength training into your routine, aiming for at least 30 minutes of moderate activity most days of the week.

4. Eat a Liver-Friendly Diet

A healthy, balanced diet plays a crucial role in supporting liver function, especially when dealing with chronic stress. A diet rich in antioxidants, fiber, and anti-inflammatory foods helps to combat oxidative stress, reduce inflammation, and improve liver detoxification. Consider incorporating foods like leafy greens, berries, cruciferous vegetables (such as broccoli and kale), and healthy fats from sources like olive oil and avocados.

Avoid processed foods, excessive sugar, and alcohol, as these can exacerbate liver strain and inflammation. Supplements such as milk thistle, turmeric, and dandelion root can also provide additional liver support and aid in detoxification.

5. Seek Professional Help When Needed

If you find that stress is overwhelming or leading to symptoms of liver dysfunction, don't hesitate to seek professional help. A licensed therapist or counselor can help you manage stress and emotional health. Additionally, if you're experiencing symptoms of liver disease, it's essential to consult a healthcare provider who can guide you on the appropriate steps for diagnosis and treatment.

Stress and emotional health are key factors in maintaining liver health and promoting healing. Understanding the direct link between chronic stress, liver function, and the gut-liver axis provides invaluable insights into how we can take charge of our health. By managing stress through lifestyle changes such as mindfulness, exercise, sleep, and diet, we can significantly reduce the burden on the liver and promote healing.

A holistic approach that addresses both physical and emotional well-being is vital for liver recovery. Taking action now to reduce stress and enhance emotional health will not only support liver function but improve overall quality of life.

Mindfulness and Meditation for Liver Health

Mindfulness and meditation are powerful practices that have gained widespread recognition for their ability to improve mental and physical well-being. But did you know that these practices can also play a crucial role in maintaining liver health? The liver, being a vital organ, is responsible for detoxification, metabolism, and other essential functions that impact the body's overall balance. Stress, poor mental health, and anxiety can put additional strain on the liver, making it harder for the organ to perform its vital duties. Mindfulness and meditation can help reduce this burden by addressing the root cause: stress.

How Stress Affects the Liver

In today's fast-paced world, stress has become a constant companion. The liver, in its role as a detoxifier, is often overburdened by the constant release of toxins, many of which come from stress hormones like cortisol. When the body is stressed, it goes into "fight or flight" mode, activating the release of these hormones that prepare us to either face danger or escape from it. While this response is useful in short bursts, chronic stress can lead to harmful consequences.

Prolonged stress causes the liver to work overtime, processing toxins and maintaining blood sugar levels. This increases the risk of liver diseases such as fatty liver disease, cirrhosis, and hepatitis. Moreover, stress can worsen inflammation in the liver, leading to greater damage.

Mindfulness and Meditation: A Holistic Approach to Liver Health

Mindfulness is the practice of staying present in the moment without judgment. It involves being aware of your thoughts, feelings, and surroundings with full attention. Meditation, on the other hand, is a technique that can help calm the mind and create a state of focused relaxation. When combined, mindfulness and meditation can be powerful tools in managing stress, which indirectly supports liver health.

Studies have shown that mindfulness and meditation can lower cortisol levels, reduce inflammation, and improve emotional well-being. By calming the nervous system and creating a sense of relaxation, these practices help the liver function optimally. Furthermore, when you're mindful, you are more attuned to your body's signals, which allows you to recognize early signs of stress, liver discomfort, or other health issues.

The Science Behind Mindfulness and Liver Health

Research has demonstrated that chronic stress can affect the liver's ability to detoxify, store nutrients, and regulate fat. For instance, stress-related conditions like insulin resistance, high cholesterol, and fatty liver disease have been linked to prolonged emotional distress. In contrast, mindfulness and meditation have been shown to reduce the production of stress hormones and improve liver function.

In one study, participants who practiced mindfulness meditation regularly showed significant reductions in inflammation markers. These results were especially encouraging for people with chronic liver diseases, where inflammation plays a central role in disease progression.

Mindfulness Practices for Liver Health

There are several types of mindfulness practices you can incorporate into your daily routine to support liver health:

1. **Body Scan Meditation** – This involves mentally scanning each part of your body from head to toe, paying close attention to areas of tension or discomfort. It helps you

become more aware of physical sensations and reduces stress.

2. **Mindful Breathing** – Sit quietly and pay attention to your breath. Notice the rise and fall of your abdomen as you breathe in and out. Focus your attention on each breath, which can help calm your nervous system and reduce stress.

3. **Loving-Kindness Meditation** – This involves focusing on sending positive thoughts and well wishes to yourself and others. It can increase feelings of compassion and reduce negative emotions, lowering overall stress levels.

4. **Mindful Eating** – Pay close attention to what and how you eat. By being present during meals, you help reduce stress related to food choices and digestion, both of which impact liver health.

Incorporating Meditation into Your Life

Meditation is another tool that can complement mindfulness. There are various forms of meditation that can specifically help with stress reduction:

1. **Guided Meditation** – A teacher or an app leads you through a relaxation process, helping you focus and release tension.

2. **Breathing Meditation** – Focus on your breath, slowly inhaling and exhaling. This promotes relaxation and lowers cortisol levels.

3. **Zen Meditation (Zazen)** – A seated practice where you focus on the breath while observing your thoughts without attachment. This can help clear the mind and reduce overall mental clutter.

Incorporating mindfulness and meditation into your daily routine can greatly improve your mental health and, by extension, your liver health. Stress management is key to reducing the burden on the liver and preventing or managing liver diseases. Start small and gradually build up your practice. Even just five minutes of mindful breathing every day can make a world of difference in your liver health and overall well-being.

Simple Practices to Lower Stress Levels

Stress is an unavoidable part of life, but how we handle it can make a world of difference to our overall health, particularly to the health of our liver. The liver is the body's detox powerhouse, and when it's overwhelmed by stress, it struggles to perform its functions effectively. Over time, this can lead to liver conditions such as fatty liver, cirrhosis, or inflammation. To ensure your liver stays healthy, it is essential to find simple yet effective ways to manage stress.

Why Lowering Stress Is Essential for Liver Health

Stress triggers a complex chain of reactions in the body. When we experience stress, the body releases stress hormones, such as cortisol, which prepare us to face immediate threats. This is the fight-or-flight response in action. However, prolonged or chronic stress keeps the body in this heightened state, and this constant demand on the body can cause serious harm, including liver damage.

Cortisol increases blood sugar and fat, both of which put stress on the liver. Additionally, stress causes inflammation throughout the body, including in the liver, which is a known precursor to liver diseases. Lowering stress levels can therefore play a vital role in preventing liver issues and improving overall well-being.

1. Physical Exercise to Relieve Stress

Exercise is one of the most effective ways to reduce stress. Regular physical activity stimulates the production of endorphins, the body's natural mood elevators. These neurotransmitters can reduce the effects of stress, promote relaxation, and help lower cortisol levels.

You don't need to run a marathon to see the benefits. Even light exercise, such as walking, swimming, or yoga, can provide significant stress relief. Aim for at least 30 minutes of moderate activity, several times a week. The key is consistency.

Exercise also helps maintain a healthy weight and prevents the accumulation of fat in the liver, reducing the risk of fatty liver disease.

2. Proper Sleep Hygiene

Sleep is crucial for stress management. When you don't get enough sleep, your body becomes more prone to stress, and cortisol levels rise. This makes it harder for the liver to detoxify and carry out its essential functions. By prioritizing sleep, you allow your body and liver to rest and repair.

To improve your sleep quality, maintain a regular sleep schedule, create a peaceful environment for sleeping, and avoid caffeine or heavy meals before bed. Sleep hygiene is an important component in managing stress levels.

3. Nutrition and a Healthy Diet

What you eat plays a significant role in how your body responds to stress. Diets rich in whole foods like fruits, vegetables, and lean proteins support liver health and help reduce the effects of stress. Avoid processed foods and excessive sugar, as they can increase inflammation and make it harder for your liver to function properly.

A balanced diet with anti-inflammatory foods, such as leafy greens, turmeric, and fatty fish, can support both mental and physical well-being. These foods nourish the liver and help to counteract the stress that burdens it.

4. Social Connection and Support

Humans are social creatures, and having a strong social network can significantly reduce stress. Spending time with loved ones, sharing experiences, or even seeking professional counseling can help you manage emotional stress more effectively.

Engaging in social activities or joining groups where you can talk openly about your feelings is an excellent way to relieve stress and ensure that your mental state remains healthy, thereby supporting your liver's function.

5. Time Management and Setting Boundaries

One of the biggest sources of stress is feeling overwhelmed by responsibilities. Learning to manage your time effectively can reduce this strain. Break large tasks into smaller, manageable steps, and prioritize what's most important.

Additionally, it's important to set boundaries. Learn to say no when necessary and delegate tasks. By managing your time and commitments wisely, you reduce stress and create more space for relaxation and recovery.

6. Mindful Breathing and Relaxation Techniques

Mindful breathing is a simple yet powerful way to calm the mind and lower stress levels. Deep breathing exercises can slow down your heart rate, lower cortisol, and activate the body's relaxation response. You can practice mindful breathing anywhere—whether at home, in traffic, or at work.

To practice mindful breathing:

- Sit or lie down in a comfortable position.
- Close your eyes and take a deep breath in through your nose.
- Hold for a few seconds, and then slowly exhale through your mouth.
- Repeat this cycle for several minutes.

Lowering stress is one of the most impactful things you can do to protect your liver. Simple practices, such as regular exercise, healthy sleep habits, proper nutrition, and mindful breathing, can have a profound effect on both your mental and liver health. Take a few minutes each day to engage in these stress-reducing practices, and you'll soon feel the difference in your overall health and well-being.

Breathing Techniques to Calm the Mind and Heal the Body

Breathing is something we all do naturally, but it's also something we can consciously control. Breathing exercises have been used for centuries as tools for healing, relaxation, and stress management. The ability to slow down and regulate your breath can be a powerful way to calm your mind, reduce stress, and even promote liver health.

Why Breathing Matters for Liver Health

The liver is sensitive to stress and inflammation, which can be caused by rapid, shallow breathing associated with anxiety and stress. Shallow breathing signals the body to remain in a state of alertness, which keeps stress hormones like cortisol elevated. Chronic high levels of cortisol can contribute to liver dysfunction.

On the other hand, controlled, deep breathing can lower cortisol levels and activate the body's parasympathetic nervous system, promoting a state of relaxation. By practicing specific breathing techniques, you can reduce stress, improve circulation, and support your liver's ability to detoxify and perform its vital functions.

Types of Breathing Techniques

1. Diaphragmatic Breathing (Belly Breathing)

Diaphragmatic breathing involves engaging the diaphragm to take slow, deep breaths. This type of breathing increases oxygen intake, stimulates the vagus nerve (which helps lower heart rate and blood pressure), and calms the nervous system.

To practice diaphragmatic breathing:

- Sit or lie down in a relaxed position.
- Place one hand on your chest and the other on your abdomen.
- Take a slow, deep breath in through your nose, allowing your abdomen to rise as you fill your lungs.

- Exhale slowly through your mouth, letting your abdomen fall.
- Focus on the rise and fall of your abdomen, not your chest.

2. 4-7-8 Breathing Technique

This technique is designed to calm the mind and body quickly. It's simple and effective, helping you to fall into a state of relaxation within a few minutes.

To practice 4-7-8 breathing:

- Inhale quietly through your nose for a count of four.
- Hold your breath for a count of seven.
- Exhale completely and audibly through your mouth for a count of eight.
- Repeat this cycle for several minutes.

3. Alternate Nostril Breathing (Nadi Shodhana)

Alternate nostril breathing is a yogic practice that balances the flow of energy in the body, calms the mind, and promotes relaxation.

To practice alternate nostril breathing:

- Sit comfortably and close your right nostril with your right thumb.
- Inhale deeply through your left nostril.
- Close your left nostril with your right ring finger, and release the right nostril.
- Exhale through the right nostril.
- Inhale through the right nostril.
- Close the right nostril and release the left nostril.
- Exhale through the left nostril.

- Repeat for several minutes.

Breathing techniques are an accessible and effective way to reduce stress, promote liver health, and achieve mental clarity. By incorporating these simple practices into your daily routine, you can help lower your stress levels, calm your mind, and support your liver's detoxification process. Remember, the way you breathe can either increase or decrease your stress—take control and practice mindful breathing to heal both the mind and the body.

The Role of Positive Emotions in Liver Health

The liver, an extraordinary organ, is often seen as the body's main detoxifier. But, while physical factors such as diet, exercise, and environmental toxins often dominate discussions of liver health, it's important to recognize the lesser-known role that emotions play in the health of this vital organ. Positive emotions—such as joy, gratitude, and love—affect the body in ways we are only beginning to understand, influencing everything from our mental state to the functioning of vital organs, including the liver.

Emotions are intricately connected to the body's internal systems. Stress, anger, and frustration have long been recognized as contributing to various diseases, especially those related to the liver. However, positive emotions like joy and gratitude also have a profound effect. These emotions can help regulate liver health, boosting its ability to detoxify and protect against damage.

Let's begin by considering how emotions manifest physically. When we experience strong, negative emotions, such as anger or fear, the body responds by releasing certain hormones like cortisol and adrenaline. These chemicals, designed to help us respond to stress, have been shown to negatively affect liver function. Over time, chronic emotional stress can lead to inflammation, which is one of the primary contributors to liver diseases like fatty liver, cirrhosis, and even liver cancer.

On the other hand, positive emotions can help balance out the stress hormones. When we experience feelings of joy or gratitude, our body releases oxytocin, serotonin, and endorphins, the body's "feel-good" hormones. These chemicals support a state of relaxation and well-being, enabling the liver to function more efficiently. They also reduce the level of cortisol, allowing the body to lower stress levels, promote healing, and repair any damage to the liver.

There is scientific evidence showing the connection between emotional well-being and liver health. For instance, a study in the *Journal of Hepatology* found that patients with liver diseases who reported higher levels of emotional well-being had better overall health outcomes than those with higher levels of stress. The liver is a resilient organ, and when supported by positive emotions, it has the capacity to regenerate and heal itself, even in cases of liver damage.

One aspect of this connection is the liver's role in detoxification. The liver filters toxins from the blood and breaks down harmful substances. Emotional states can either facilitate or hinder this process. When the body is in a relaxed, positive state, it can perform detoxification more effectively. The opposite is true in a state of chronic stress or emotional turmoil, where the liver may be overburdened and less capable of eliminating toxins.

As we age, the liver's ability to regenerate and detoxify naturally declines. The good news is that positive emotions can help slow down this process. By reducing emotional stress and embracing joy, gratitude, and love, individuals can support their liver in staying healthier longer. There is no magic bullet for liver health, but emotional well-being certainly plays an important role.

It is also worth noting the connection between emotions and lifestyle choices. People who experience happiness and joy tend to take better care of themselves. They are more likely to eat healthier foods, engage in regular physical activity, and avoid harmful substances. In contrast, individuals experiencing negative emotions may turn to unhealthy coping mechanisms such as smoking, excessive drinking, or overeating. These behaviors can further contribute to liver damage. Therefore, cultivating positive emotions directly impacts the choices we make regarding our health.

In conclusion, while the liver is responsible for many vital functions, emotional health has an undeniable impact on its ability to function well. Positive emotions not only reduce stress but also improve the body's natural healing processes, giving the liver the support it needs to stay healthy. As you move forward in your journey to liver health, remember that fostering an attitude of joy, gratitude, and love can go a long way in supporting your body's most vital detoxifying organ.

How Gratitude and Joy Can Benefit Your Liver

Gratitude and joy—simple, yet powerful emotions—have been shown to play a significant role in overall health, especially when it comes to liver function. As we all know, the liver is a crucial organ for detoxification, and its health directly impacts our overall well-being. But the relationship between emotional states like gratitude and joy and liver health may not be as widely recognized. Let's delve into how these positive emotions help maintain and improve liver health, while also boosting general vitality.

The Physiological Mechanism of Gratitude and Joy

To understand how gratitude and joy benefit the liver, we must first take a look at how these emotions influence the body's systems. Emotions, particularly those that evoke positive feelings, trigger a cascade of biochemical responses that can either promote or hinder bodily functions. Gratitude and joy trigger the release of key hormones such as oxytocin, serotonin, and dopamine—often called the "feel-good" hormones. These chemicals have the ability to lower stress levels and promote a sense of calm and contentment, both of which have a direct impact on liver health.

When we experience joy or gratitude, these hormones act as natural antidotes to the harmful effects of stress hormones like cortisol. Cortisol, the hormone released during stress, can cause inflammation, inhibit the liver's detoxification processes, and weaken the immune system. On the other hand, positive emotions like joy and gratitude help reverse this effect. They help relax the nervous system, reduce stress, and provide an overall sense of well-being. This allows the liver to function more efficiently, promoting detoxification and aiding in regeneration.

Gratitude has been shown to improve general emotional well-being. Studies indicate that individuals who practice gratitude regularly have lower levels of cortisol and improved cardiovascular health. The liver, being a crucial organ for detoxification, benefits when cortisol is kept in check. In addition, gratitude fosters a positive mindset that encourages healthier lifestyle habits, such as better food choices, regular physical activity, and lower rates of substance abuse. These healthy choices directly benefit the liver by reducing the burden on the organ and supporting its optimal function.

Stress Reduction and Liver Health

As we've already discussed, the liver plays a key role in detoxifying the body by breaking down harmful substances and toxins. Chronic stress, however, can overload the liver and prevent it from performing this task effectively. By promoting joy and gratitude, you reduce the stress that can inhibit liver function. Positive emotions help relax the body, improve digestion, and reduce inflammation, making the liver's job easier.

A joyful, grateful heart leads to lower levels of anxiety and stress, which can otherwise cause or exacerbate liver-related conditions such as fatty liver disease, cirrhosis, and liver inflammation. These emotional states make it easier for the liver to heal itself, as it is not constantly dealing with the negative effects of stress hormones. This provides a sense of balance within the body, ensuring the liver remains resilient and capable of performing its vital detoxification processes.

Joy and Liver Regeneration

One of the liver's most remarkable characteristics is its ability to regenerate. The liver can heal itself after injury, whether from physical damage or metabolic stress. However, for this regeneration to occur, the body must be in an optimal state, free from chronic stress and negative emotions. By practicing gratitude and engaging in joyful activities, you are essentially setting the stage for your liver to repair itself.

Joyful experiences—whether it's spending time with loved ones, engaging in a hobby, or even laughing—create a state of relaxation that supports liver regeneration. In fact, research shows that laughter, which is often associated with joy, helps improve circulation, reduces stress, and boosts immune function. These effects enhance the liver's ability to detoxify, regenerate, and protect against diseases.

Practical Tips to Foster Gratitude and Joy

Now that we understand the powerful effects of gratitude and joy on liver health, let's look at some practical ways to incorporate these emotions into daily life:

1. **Practice Gratitude Daily**: Take a moment each day to reflect on the things you're grateful for. This can be as simple as acknowledging the support of loved ones, the beauty of nature, or your overall health. Journaling your thoughts of gratitude is an excellent way to reinforce these positive feelings.

2. **Engage in Joyful Activities**: Whether it's dancing, singing, gardening, or spending time with friends, prioritize activities that bring you happiness. The more joy you experience, the greater the positive impact on your liver and overall health.

3. **Meditation and Deep Breathing**: These relaxation techniques can help reduce stress and boost feelings of gratitude and joy. Even a few minutes a day can make a big difference in liver function.

4. **Surround Yourself with Positive People**: The people you interact with greatly influence your emotional state. Seek out those who uplift you and support your well-being.

By incorporating these habits into your life, you will not only enhance your emotional well-being but also provide vital support to your liver, helping it to perform its detoxifying role more effectively.

Releasing Emotional Toxins for Better Health

We often hear about physical toxins—heavy metals, pesticides, and pollutants—and the damage they can do to our bodies. However, one type of toxin that is rarely discussed is emotional toxins. These are the negative emotions and unresolved emotional traumas that can accumulate over time, affecting both our mental and physical health. Just as the liver works to filter out physical toxins, it also has a role in managing emotional toxins. Releasing these emotional burdens is key to improving liver health and overall well-being.

Emotional Toxins and Their Impact on the Liver

Emotions such as anger, guilt, fear, and sadness can be likened to toxins. When these emotions are repressed or left unresolved, they create internal "blockages" that affect both the mind and body. These negative emotions can manifest physically, leading to chronic stress, inflammation, and other conditions that tax the liver. The liver, as a detoxifying organ, is highly sensitive to these emotional toxins. When it is overwhelmed by emotional stress, its ability to process physical toxins and regenerate is diminished.

One of the most notable emotional toxins that negatively impacts the liver is chronic stress. Stress is one of the leading contributors to liver disease. When we are constantly under stress, our bodies release stress hormones like cortisol, which cause inflammation and harm the liver over time. Additionally, unresolved emotional trauma can cause a person to adopt unhealthy coping mechanisms, such as overeating, drinking, or smoking, all of which add more strain on the liver.

How to Release Emotional Toxins

Just as it's important to remove physical toxins through a healthy diet, exercise, and detoxification practices, it's equally essential to release emotional toxins. This can be done through several strategies that promote emotional healing:

1. **Emotional Expression**: Bottling up emotions can lead to long-term harm. It's important to express how you feel, whether it's through talking to a trusted friend or therapist, writing in a journal, or practicing creative outlets like art or music. These expressions help release pent-up emotional energy and relieve emotional burden.

2. **Forgiveness**: Holding onto resentment, anger, or guilt not only harms emotional health but can have physical consequences as well. By practicing forgiveness—whether it's forgiving others or yourself—you remove emotional toxins and allow your liver and body to heal.

3. **Mindfulness and Meditation**: These practices help center the mind and release the grip of negative emotions. Meditation allows you to observe your emotions without judgment and gently release them, promoting emotional healing and liver health.

4. **Breathwork**: Deep breathing exercises help calm the nervous system and clear emotional blockages. By focusing on your breath and exhaling deeply, you can release negative emotions and reduce stress.

5. **Physical Exercise**: Physical movement, whether through yoga, walking, or other forms of exercise, helps release pent-up emotions. Exercise promotes the production of endorphins, which can counteract emotional toxins and support emotional well-being.

The Healing Power of Emotional Release

When emotional toxins are released, the body is able to function more harmoniously. The liver, in particular, becomes less burdened and more capable of carrying out its important functions. By reducing stress, releasing repressed emotions, and practicing emotional healing, you allow the liver to detoxify more effectively, regenerate more efficiently, and maintain its vital role in overall health.

Chapter 9: Detoxing the Liver Safely and Effectively

The liver, the body's natural detoxifier, plays an essential role in cleaning toxins and waste materials from the body. While it is designed to process and remove harmful substances, our modern lifestyles, filled with poor diets, environmental toxins, and stress, can sometimes overwhelm the liver's natural detoxification processes. This is why many people turn to liver detox programs to cleanse their bodies and enhance their liver's functionality.

However, detoxing the liver requires careful planning and knowledge to avoid harming the organ instead of helping it. In this section, we will explore how to detox the liver safely and effectively.

Understanding the Liver's Detoxification Process

The liver's job is to filter and break down toxins, chemicals, and waste products so they can be eliminated from the body. It works tirelessly to remove substances like alcohol, medications, pollutants, and metabolic byproducts. The liver accomplishes this through two main phases:

- **Phase 1** involves the transformation of fat-soluble toxins into water-soluble compounds. Enzymes break down these substances, making them easier to remove from the body.
- **Phase 2** is the conjugation phase, where the liver attaches small molecules (like sulfate or glucuronic acid) to the toxins, which helps them become even more water-soluble for easier excretion through bile or urine.

Maintaining the liver's health is critical to its detoxifying function. Without a properly functioning liver, toxins can build up, leading to a range of health issues like fatigue, skin problems, digestive disturbances, and more severe conditions like fatty liver disease.

Safe Liver Detox: Why a Holistic Approach Is Necessary

While there are many liver detox supplements and cleanses on the market, not all of them are safe or effective. Some cleanses can flood the liver with additional toxins or overwhelm its natural detox systems, leading to more harm than good. The best way to detox the liver is through a combination of dietary changes, lifestyle improvements, and natural supplements that support liver function.

1. **Hydration**: One of the most important factors for liver detoxification is staying hydrated. Water helps the liver flush out toxins and supports the kidneys in removing waste. Aim for at least 8-10 glasses of water a day.

2. **Whole Foods**: Eating a balanced diet rich in fruits, vegetables, lean proteins, and whole grains provides the liver with essential nutrients to support its detox processes. Certain foods like cruciferous vegetables (broccoli, cabbage, cauliflower) and garlic contain compounds that stimulate liver enzymes and help remove toxins.

3. **Healthy Fats**: While many detox programs advocate for fat-free diets, healthy fats are essential for liver health. Omega-3 fatty acids found in fish, flaxseeds, and walnuts help reduce inflammation in the liver and promote its natural detox processes.

4. **Liver-Supportive Supplements**: Milk thistle, dandelion root, and turmeric are all herbs that support liver function and help the body remove toxins. These herbs contain antioxidants and anti-inflammatory compounds that may aid liver repair and detoxification.

5. **Avoiding Toxins**: Limiting alcohol, processed foods, and exposure to environmental toxins (such as cigarette smoke, pesticides, and chemicals in cleaning products) is crucial for maintaining liver health. Giving your liver time to rest by avoiding alcohol and other harmful substances is vital during any detox process.

How to Do a Liver Detox Safely

- **Consult a Healthcare Provider**: Before beginning any liver detox program, especially if you have a liver condition (like fatty liver disease or hepatitis), it's essential to consult a healthcare professional. They can guide you on the safest approach and ensure the detox methods won't interfere with any ongoing treatments or medications.

- **Avoid Extreme Detox Diets**: Quick-fix detox programs, such as juice cleanses or extreme fasting, may do more harm than good. The liver already works hard to detoxify the body, and extreme diets can place additional stress on it. Instead, aim for gradual lifestyle changes and a balanced approach.

- **Monitor Your Health**: During any liver detox, pay attention to how your body responds. Mild symptoms like fatigue or mild digestive discomfort are common during detox, but severe symptoms like nausea, headaches, or dizziness may indicate that the process is too intense or that your body is struggling to keep up.

By incorporating these practices into your routine, you can effectively and safely support liver detoxification and improve your overall liver health.

Liver Detox Programs: What You Need to Know

Liver detox programs are widely advertised as quick solutions to cleanse the liver and rejuvenate health. However, it's essential to approach these programs with caution, understanding the potential benefits and risks involved.

What Are Liver Detox Programs?

A liver detox program typically involves a combination of dietary changes, herbal supplements, fasting, and lifestyle modifications designed to support the liver's natural detoxification abilities. The goal of such programs is to enhance liver function, remove accumulated toxins, and promote better overall health.

These programs are available in many forms, including commercial detox kits, fasting protocols, and natural herbal remedies. Some may recommend cutting out processed foods, alcohol, and caffeine, while others may suggest a juice cleanse or a restrictive diet for a set period.

Types of Liver Detox Programs

1. **Juice Cleanses**: These programs typically involve consuming only juices made from fruits and vegetables for a certain number of days. They are designed to give the

digestive system a break while flooding the body with nutrients. However, while juices provide vitamins and antioxidants, they lack essential proteins and fats necessary for liver repair.

2. **Herbal Liver Cleanses**: These programs use herbs like milk thistle, dandelion root, and turmeric to help stimulate the liver's detoxification process. These herbs are thought to support liver function by providing antioxidants, reducing inflammation, and promoting bile production.

3. **Fasting Programs**: Intermittent fasting or periodic fasting is another approach used in liver detox programs. The theory is that fasting allows the liver to focus on detoxifying instead of processing food, while also promoting autophagy (the body's natural cell-repair process).

4. **Diet-Based Liver Detox**: A more balanced approach to liver detox involves adopting a diet rich in liver-supporting foods, such as cruciferous vegetables, garlic, ginger, turmeric, and green tea. This is often a more sustainable approach that emphasizes long-term lifestyle changes.

What You Should Expect from a Liver Detox Program

When you start a liver detox program, you may experience a variety of symptoms as your body adjusts to the changes. Here's what you can expect:

- **Increased Energy**: As your liver clears out toxins, you may notice an improvement in energy levels and better overall vitality.

- **Digestive Changes**: A liver detox may improve digestion, reduce bloating, and promote regular bowel movements as the liver becomes more efficient at eliminating waste.

- **Flu-Like Symptoms**: Some people may experience headaches, nausea, or mild flu-like symptoms during the detox process. This is a common sign of the body eliminating toxins, but if symptoms persist or worsen, consult a doctor.

- **Clearer Skin**: Since the liver is responsible for processing waste, you may notice improvements in skin conditions such as acne, eczema, or psoriasis.

It's essential to approach liver detox programs as part of a long-term health strategy, not just a short-term fix. Consistency in diet, lifestyle habits, and the use of natural supplements will lead to the best outcomes.

What to Expect During a Liver Detox

While liver detox programs promise great results, it's important to know what to expect during the process. Detoxing the liver is not a quick fix, and the process may involve several stages.

Initial Symptoms of Liver Detox

- **Fatigue**: As toxins begin to leave the body, you may feel more tired than usual. This is due to the increased work your liver is doing to filter out toxins.

- **Digestive Changes**: You may experience changes in digestion, such as bloating or increased bowel movements. This can be a sign that your liver is becoming more efficient at processing waste.

- **Mood Swings**: Toxins leaving the body can sometimes affect your mood, leading to irritability or emotional ups and downs.

- **Skin Breakouts**: As the liver detoxifies, it may push toxins out through the skin, causing temporary acne or rashes.

Supporting Your Body During Detox

During the detox process, it's crucial to take steps to support your body. Make sure to:

- **Stay Hydrated**: Drink plenty of water to help flush toxins out of your system.
- **Get Rest**: Adequate sleep is essential for recovery and to help your body detox effectively.
- **Eat Liver-Supportive Foods**: Focus on a diet rich in antioxidants, vitamins, and minerals to support the liver.

While liver detox can be uncomfortable at times, the benefits of a cleaner, more efficient liver far outweigh the temporary discomforts. Be patient, stay consistent, and listen to your body's needs.

Myths vs. Facts About Liver Cleanses

Liver detox and cleansing programs have been surrounded by various myths that may confuse people looking for safe and effective ways to improve liver health. Here are a few myths and the truths behind them:

Myth 1: Liver Cleanses Are Only for People with Liver Disease

Fact: Anyone can benefit from supporting liver health, not just those with liver disease. The liver is constantly exposed to toxins and pollutants, and maintaining its health is essential for optimal functioning, whether or not a liver condition is present.

Myth 2: Extreme Fasting is the Best Way to Detox the Liver

Fact: While fasting may provide short-term benefits, extreme fasting can be harmful. The liver needs a balanced intake of nutrients to detox effectively, and depriving the body of food can actually stress the liver and hinder detoxification.

Myth 3: All Liver Detox Programs Are Safe

Fact: Not all detox programs are created equal. Some liver detox programs can involve harsh chemicals or extreme practices that may harm the liver rather than help it. Always choose a safe, scientifically backed approach.

Myth 4: Liver Detox Programs Provide Instant Results

Fact: Detoxing the liver is a gradual process that requires time and consistent effort. Instant results are unrealistic, and true liver detoxification is achieved through long-term lifestyle changes.

Risks and Benefits of Detoxing

Detoxing the liver offers a range of benefits, but it also comes with some risks if done improperly. Here, we'll break down both the benefits and the potential risks of liver detox programs.

Benefits of Detoxing the Liver

- **Improved Energy**: A detoxified liver can increase energy levels and reduce fatigue.
- **Better Digestion**: A cleaner liver promotes better digestion and nutrient absorption.
- **Clearer Skin**: As the liver detoxifies, your skin may clear up, reducing acne and other skin issues.
- **Reduced Inflammation**: A healthy liver can help reduce systemic inflammation, which is linked to various chronic diseases.

Risks of Detoxing the Liver

- **Uncomfortable Symptoms**: Detoxing can cause mild to moderate symptoms like fatigue, headaches, and digestive issues.
- **Nutrient Deficiencies**: Some extreme detox diets may lack essential nutrients, leading to deficiencies.
- **Overloading the Liver**: Some detox programs may overwhelm the liver, especially if they are too aggressive or require fasting.

Liver detoxification is beneficial when done correctly. By understanding the risks, debunking myths, and following a safe, balanced approach, you can effectively support your liver's health and overall wellness. Always consult with a healthcare professional before starting any detox program, especially if you have pre-existing health conditions.

Gentle Detox Methods for Beginners

Detoxification, or the process of removing toxins from the body, can seem like an overwhelming concept, especially for beginners. However, it doesn't have to be complicated or extreme. As a matter of fact, gentle detox methods are often the most effective and sustainable way to support your liver and overall health without causing unnecessary stress or discomfort.

The liver is our body's main detoxification organ. It works tirelessly to filter toxins, break down harmful substances, and eliminate waste products. However, due to modern lifestyles, environmental toxins, poor diet, and stress, the liver can become overloaded. When this happens, it can affect the body's ability to eliminate waste efficiently, leading to fatigue, skin issues, digestive problems, and even more serious health concerns.

Here, we'll explore some simple, beginner-friendly detox methods that allow your liver to do its job while supporting overall health. These methods are designed to be easy to integrate into daily life without the need for drastic dietary changes or extreme fasting. The goal is to gently encourage the body's natural detoxification processes.

1. Hydration: The Foundation of Detox

The first and most essential step in any detox plan is proper hydration. Water helps flush out toxins and waste products through the kidneys, and it's crucial for keeping the liver functioning efficiently. It is important to consume enough water to keep your body hydrated and support the removal of waste. As a general rule, aim for 8-10 glasses of water a day, though individual needs may vary based on age, activity level, and climate.

In addition to plain water, herbal teas such as dandelion root, milk thistle, and ginger tea can support liver health and enhance detoxification. These herbs have been traditionally used for their detoxifying properties, helping the liver process toxins more efficiently. Avoid sugary drinks, sodas, and excessive caffeine, as they can burden the liver.

2. Eating Whole, Natural Foods

A gentle detox begins with what you put into your body. Whole, natural foods like fruits, vegetables, lean proteins, and whole grains provide the nutrients needed to nourish and cleanse your body. Fiber-rich foods are particularly important for detoxification, as they help eliminate waste through the digestive system.

Focus on including plenty of fresh, seasonal vegetables such as leafy greens (spinach, kale, and swiss chard), cruciferous vegetables (broccoli, cauliflower, and cabbage), and root vegetables (carrots, beets, and sweet potatoes). These vegetables support liver function and provide antioxidants that protect the liver from oxidative stress.

Fruits like berries, apples, and citrus fruits are rich in vitamins and antioxidants that help detoxify the body. Citrus fruits, in particular, are known for their high vitamin C content, which is a powerful antioxidant that supports liver function and boosts the immune system.

3. Eliminating Processed Foods and Toxins

A significant part of a gentle detox is eliminating the foods and substances that burden the liver. Processed foods, refined sugars, alcohol, and artificial chemicals are difficult for the liver to process and can lead to a buildup of toxins in the body. These foods often lack essential nutrients, and instead, they may contain harmful additives, preservatives, and unhealthy fats.

Start by reducing your intake of packaged foods, fast foods, and sugary snacks. Instead, opt for homemade meals made with fresh ingredients. This is an excellent way to improve your liver health and avoid the chemicals found in processed food.

4. Gentle Exercise: Sweating it Out

Exercise is an effective and natural way to support detoxification. When you move your body, you increase blood circulation and stimulate the lymphatic system, which is responsible for removing toxins. Sweating also helps eliminate toxins through the skin.

Engage in gentle activities like walking, swimming, or yoga. These forms of exercise are low-impact but highly effective at boosting circulation and supporting the liver. Aim for at least 30 minutes of physical activity each day. Gentle exercises are not only good for your liver, but they also help reduce stress, improve mood, and increase energy levels.

5. Sleep and Stress Management

Detoxification doesn't just happen during the day; it continues while you sleep. Adequate sleep is essential for the body's natural detoxification process. During sleep, the liver is able to focus on cleaning and processing toxins that have accumulated throughout the day.

In addition to sleep, managing stress is crucial for a successful detox. Chronic stress can impair liver function and increase the production of toxic substances in the body. Practice relaxation techniques such as deep breathing, meditation, or journaling to help keep your stress levels in check.

6. Herbal Supplements and Liver Support

Certain herbs and supplements can assist the liver in its detoxification processes. Milk thistle, dandelion root, and turmeric are particularly well-known for their liver-supportive properties. These herbs can be taken in the form of tea or supplements, but always consult with a healthcare provider before starting any new supplement regimen, especially if you have preexisting conditions.

Simple Liver-Friendly Detox Plans

Now that we've covered the basics of gentle detox, let's look at some simple liver-friendly detox plans. These plans are designed to gradually support your liver without overwhelming your body or requiring drastic changes.

1. The 3-Day Liver Detox Plan

This beginner-friendly detox plan is designed to jumpstart your liver's cleansing process and help you feel revitalized. It focuses on hydrating, eating whole foods, and eliminating common toxins.

Day 1: Hydration and Cleanse

- Start your day with warm water and lemon to stimulate digestion.
- Drink herbal teas like dandelion root or milk thistle throughout the day to support liver function.

- Eat light meals made from fresh vegetables, whole grains, and lean proteins. Avoid heavy meats, dairy, and processed foods.
- Drink plenty of water, at least 8 glasses, throughout the day.
- Engage in light exercise, such as a brisk walk, to help boost circulation.

Day 2: Focus on Fiber and Antioxidants

- Eat fiber-rich meals that include lots of fresh vegetables, fruits, and whole grains. Foods like spinach, kale, sweet potatoes, and berries are particularly beneficial.
- Include healthy fats like avocado, olive oil, and nuts to support the liver's ability to break down toxins.
- Avoid alcohol, caffeine, and refined sugars.
- Drink detox-friendly teas and hydrate with water.
- Engage in moderate physical activity, such as yoga or swimming, to promote circulation and sweating.

Day 3: Rest and Nourish

- Focus on foods that are easy to digest, like soups or smoothies made from fruits and vegetables.
- Continue to hydrate with water and herbal teas.
- Take time for relaxation, such as deep breathing or meditation, to help manage stress.
- Avoid overexerting yourself, and let your body rest while it continues to detoxify.

2. The 7-Day Detox Plan

A 7-day detox plan is slightly more intensive but still gentle and supportive. This plan encourages whole foods, gentle exercise, and a break from processed foods to give the liver a deeper cleanse.

Day 1-3: Hydration and Nutrition

- Focus on hydrating with water and herbal teas.
- Eat whole, plant-based meals, including plenty of leafy greens, cruciferous vegetables, and fruits like apples and berries.
- Limit your intake of animal proteins and dairy products.
- Add liver-supportive foods like turmeric, garlic, and beets to your meals.
- Take walks and engage in light activities to keep the body active.

Day 4-5: Cleanse and Rest

- Continue to avoid processed foods, alcohol, and refined sugars.
- Include more high-antioxidant foods, such as green tea, berries, and dark leafy greens.
- Begin to incorporate restorative activities like meditation or journaling to reduce stress.
- Engage in light-to-moderate exercise, such as walking or gentle yoga.

Day 6-7: Final Rest and Rejuvenate

- Continue eating simple, nourishing foods, avoiding processed snacks and heavy meals.
- Focus on hydration, herbal teas, and restful sleep.
- Take time to relax and allow your body to naturally eliminate toxins.

How to Safely Introduce Detox Foods into Your Diet

Introducing detox foods into your diet can seem daunting, especially if you're new to detoxification. However, with a bit of planning and patience, you can gradually incorporate these foods into your meals in a way that supports your liver and overall health.

1. Start Slow

Begin by incorporating one or two detox foods into your diet each week. For example, you might start with adding a cup of dandelion tea or a serving of leafy greens to your meals. Don't feel the need to make dramatic changes overnight. Instead, focus on gradual, sustainable shifts that allow your body to adjust without overwhelming it.

2. Diversify Your Diet

The key to a successful detox is variety. Make sure you're including a wide range of detox-friendly foods, including leafy greens, cruciferous vegetables, citrus fruits, and healthy fats. For example, you could enjoy a smoothie made with spinach, kale, berries, and chia seeds or add some garlic and turmeric to your soups.

3. Combine Detox Foods with Balanced Meals

Detox foods should be a part of a balanced diet, not a replacement for all other foods. For example, a healthy detox meal could consist of grilled chicken or tofu, a serving of steamed broccoli, a sweet potato, and a drizzle of olive oil. Combining detox foods with healthy proteins, fats, and whole grains will give your body the fuel it needs while enhancing the detox process.

4. Be Mindful of Food Sensitivities

As you introduce new foods into your diet, pay attention to how your body responds. Some people may have sensitivities to certain foods like cruciferous vegetables or citrus fruits. If you notice any discomfort, it's a good idea to adjust your diet accordingly.

These beginner-friendly detox methods and plans are a gentle way to support liver health and overall wellness. By focusing on hydration, eating whole foods, and gradually incorporating liver-friendly foods, you can give your liver the support it needs without overwhelming your body. Always remember, gentle detox is a lifestyle change, not a quick fix, and patience is key to long-term success.

Cleansing Your Liver with Lifestyle Changes

Your liver is an incredible organ. It works tirelessly to filter toxins from your blood, produce bile for digestion, store essential nutrients, and even produce proteins that help with clotting. But, despite this monumental task, the liver is often overlooked when it comes to health. One of the best ways to ensure your liver remains in optimal condition is through lifestyle changes. A healthy liver is not just about avoiding toxins but also about supporting its natural detoxification process.

The liver's ability to detoxify is astonishing. It can break down harmful substances like alcohol, medications, and environmental toxins and safely remove them from your body. But the constant onslaught of these toxins—combined with poor diet, lack of exercise, and chronic stress—can leave your liver overburdened, impairing its function.

1. Nutrition: The Foundation of Liver Health

The first step in supporting your liver is a healthy diet. Your liver thrives on the nutrients you provide it through the food you consume. A nutrient-rich diet full of fruits, vegetables, whole grains, and lean proteins can help your liver perform its best. Here are some key foods and nutrients that support liver health:

Antioxidants: The Liver's Allies

Antioxidants protect your liver from oxidative stress, which can cause liver damage over time. Foods rich in antioxidants—such as berries, leafy greens, and nuts—are vital for liver detoxification. They help neutralize free radicals, which are harmful compounds that can damage liver cells.

Top Antioxidant-Rich Foods for Liver Health:

- Berries (blueberries, strawberries, and raspberries)
- Spinach, kale, and other leafy greens
- Carrots and sweet potatoes
- Walnuts and almonds

Fiber: Promoting Healthy Digestion and Detoxification

Fiber aids in digestion, which is essential for toxin elimination. It binds to waste and helps flush it out of the body, reducing the burden on the liver. A high-fiber diet also helps to regulate blood sugar levels, which is essential for those with fatty liver disease or diabetes.

High-Fiber Foods for a Healthy Liver:

- Whole grains (brown rice, quinoa, and oats)
- Beans, lentils, and peas

- Vegetables like broccoli, Brussels sprouts, and artichokes

Healthy Fats: Essential for Liver Function

Your liver needs healthy fats to function properly. Omega-3 fatty acids, found in foods like fatty fish, walnuts, and flaxseeds, have anti-inflammatory properties that help reduce liver inflammation, which is a common issue in liver disease.

Foods Rich in Omega-3 Fatty Acids:

- Fatty fish (salmon, mackerel, sardines)
- Walnuts and flaxseeds
- Chia seeds and hemp seeds

2. Hydration: Flush Out Toxins

Water is essential for nearly every function in your body, and it plays a crucial role in liver detoxification. The liver processes and eliminates waste through the kidneys, and staying hydrated ensures this process runs smoothly. Aim for at least 8 cups of water a day, more if you are physically active or live in a hot climate. Drinking lemon water, herbal teas, or coconut water can also support liver function and improve hydration.

3. Limit Alcohol and Toxins

One of the most significant ways to protect your liver is by minimizing alcohol intake. Alcohol is a toxin that is metabolized by the liver, and excessive consumption can lead to fatty liver disease, cirrhosis, and even liver cancer. Moderation is key when it comes to alcohol, and some people may benefit from eliminating alcohol altogether.

Additionally, limit exposure to environmental toxins found in household cleaners, pesticides, and industrial chemicals. These toxins can accumulate in the liver over time, making it harder for your liver to detoxify efficiently. When possible, opt for natural, non-toxic cleaning products, and choose organic produce to reduce pesticide exposure.

4. Physical Activity: Exercise for Liver Health

Regular exercise is one of the best ways to support liver function and detoxification. Physical activity helps regulate blood sugar levels, reduces liver fat, and improves circulation, all of which are crucial for liver health. Aim for at least 150 minutes of moderate-intensity exercise per week, including activities such as walking, swimming, cycling, or yoga.

5. Stress Management: Protect Your Liver from the Inside Out

Chronic stress can wreak havoc on your liver by increasing the production of cortisol, the stress hormone. High levels of cortisol can lead to inflammation, which can overtax your liver. Practices such as meditation, deep breathing, yoga, or journaling can help reduce stress and support your liver's detoxification process.

How to Support Your Liver Year-Round

Supporting your liver is not a one-time event but an ongoing process. Your liver is exposed to toxins daily, whether from food, medications, or environmental pollutants, so it's important to take steps year-round to maintain its health. Here are some ways to support your liver throughout the year:

1. Seasonal Detoxification

While your liver constantly works to detoxify your body, giving it a little extra support with a seasonal detox can be beneficial. A seasonal detox involves adopting dietary changes, reducing toxins, and supporting your liver with specific herbs and supplements.

For example, in the spring, you might focus on liver-cleansing foods like dandelion greens, artichokes, and beets, which are known to help cleanse the liver. In the fall, you can focus on immune-boosting foods like garlic, onions, and turmeric, which also have liver-supporting properties.

2. Regular Liver Cleansing

A liver cleanse doesn't necessarily mean fasting or extreme detox diets. It's about supporting the liver's natural detoxification process. Consider doing a gentle liver cleanse every few months. You can support this process by increasing your intake of water, eating liver-friendly foods, and incorporating herbs like milk thistle, dandelion root, and turmeric, which help to enhance liver function.

3. Avoid Overloading Your Liver with Toxins

Your liver doesn't only process toxins from food and drink; it also filters medications and environmental pollutants. Be mindful of how much you expose your liver to on a daily basis. Always follow your doctor's advice regarding medications, and consider switching to natural personal care products to reduce your chemical exposure. Opt for organic foods when possible to minimize pesticide intake.

4. Keep an Eye on Your Liver Health

Regular check-ups with your healthcare provider are key to monitoring liver function. Blood tests like the liver function test (LFT) can give you insight into how well your liver is working. If you have liver concerns or a family history of liver disease, make sure to keep track of your health and follow your doctor's recommendations.

Building Long-Term Liver Health Habits

Building long-term habits for liver health is essential for preventing liver disease and maintaining overall health. The following practices can help ensure your liver stays healthy for years to come.

1. Develop a Consistent Exercise Routine

Exercise isn't just for weight loss—it's a key factor in long-term liver health. Regular physical activity reduces the risk of fatty liver disease, improves liver function, and promotes the circulation of blood, which helps your liver detoxify. Aim for daily movement, whether through walking, swimming, or cycling.

2. Focus on Nutrient-Dense, Whole Foods

The foundation of long-term liver health is a nutrient-dense diet. Eating a variety of whole foods, including fruits, vegetables, lean proteins, and whole grains, provides the vitamins and minerals your liver needs to perform its vital functions. Avoid processed foods, added sugars, and trans fats, which can contribute to fatty liver disease and inflammation.

3. Make Hydration a Priority

Hydration is often overlooked, but it plays a crucial role in liver health. Chronic dehydration can hinder the liver's ability to detoxify, leading to a buildup of toxins in the body. Always make sure you are drinking enough water throughout the day. Herbal teas like milk thistle tea and dandelion tea can also support liver health.

4. Manage Your Stress Levels

Chronic stress can contribute to liver damage over time. Long-term stress increases cortisol levels, which can cause inflammation and negatively affect liver function. Adopt a healthy routine for stress management, such as meditation, mindfulness, or relaxation techniques.

5. Regular Liver Check-ups and Monitoring

As you age, it's important to keep an eye on your liver health. Regular check-ups with your healthcare provider, including blood tests and screenings for liver disease, can catch any issues early. If you have a family history of liver disease or other risk factors, make sure to stay on top of your liver health.

6. Practice Moderation with Alcohol and Medications

While occasional alcohol consumption may not harm a healthy liver, chronic heavy drinking can lead to liver disease. If you choose to drink, do so in moderation. Additionally, always follow your doctor's guidelines when it comes to medication use, as certain medications can have toxic effects on the liver.

Chapter 10: Medical and Alternative Treatments for Liver Disease

Traditional Treatments for Liver Disease

Liver disease is a serious condition, and while it may be overlooked or misunderstood, it's crucial that individuals seek medical attention early. The liver is an organ that performs essential functions like detoxification, metabolism, and nutrient storage, which is why liver disease can severely impact overall health. In this section, we will discuss traditional treatments commonly used to manage liver disease.

1. Medication

In the treatment of liver disease, medications play a key role. The choice of medications depends on the type and stage of liver disease. Some common conditions affecting the liver include Hepatitis, cirrhosis, non-alcoholic fatty liver disease (NAFLD), and alcoholic liver disease. Treatment usually aims to manage symptoms, prevent complications, and slow the progression of the disease.

- **Hepatitis Treatments:** Hepatitis is an infection that causes inflammation of the liver. Hepatitis B and C, in particular, are chronic and can lead to cirrhosis or liver cancer. Antiviral medications such as **Tenofovir** and **Entecavir** for Hepatitis B, and **Sofosbuvir**, **Ledipasvir**, and **Velpatasvir** for Hepatitis C, are commonly prescribed. These medications help to reduce the viral load, decrease liver inflammation, and prevent the virus from causing long-term damage.

- **Non-alcoholic Fatty Liver Disease (NAFLD):** NAFLD is the most common cause of liver disease in the world. Treatment mainly revolves around managing risk factors such as obesity, type 2 diabetes, and high cholesterol. Medications such as **Pioglitazone**, **Vitamin E**, and **Liraglutide** are sometimes used to reduce liver fat and inflammation. However, lifestyle changes like weight loss and regular physical activity remain the cornerstone of treatment.

- **Cirrhosis and Alcoholic Liver Disease:** For cirrhosis (scarring of the liver), treatments aim to address complications like ascites (fluid buildup in the abdomen), varices (enlarged veins in the esophagus), and encephalopathy (a decline in brain function). Medications such as **Diuretics** (to reduce fluid buildup), **Beta-blockers** (to prevent variceal bleeding), and **Lactulose** (to treat encephalopathy) are commonly used.

2. Liver Biopsy and Imaging

Traditional treatments may also involve diagnostic tools to assess the extent of liver damage. A **liver biopsy** involves taking a small tissue sample from the liver for microscopic examination to determine the degree of damage or cirrhosis. This can help doctors understand how far the disease has progressed and decide on the best course of treatment.

Other non-invasive tests like **ultrasound**, **CT scans**, and **MRI** are also frequently used to examine the liver for signs of fatty deposits, inflammation, or tumors. These imaging tests help doctors monitor the condition and determine whether additional interventions are needed.

3. Liver Transplants

A liver transplant is sometimes necessary when the liver has suffered extensive damage that cannot be reversed by medical treatments alone. Conditions like cirrhosis, end-stage liver failure, and liver cancer may lead to the need for a transplant. However, liver transplants are not a cure-all, and they come with risks and challenges, which we'll explore in more detail below.

Common Medications and Their Role in Liver Health

Medications are vital for managing liver disease, especially when the disease is chronic or advanced. Below, we will explore several classes of medications used in liver treatment, their purposes, and how they work.

1. Antiviral Medications

For individuals suffering from viral hepatitis, antiviral medications are crucial in controlling the disease and preventing it from progressing to cirrhosis or liver cancer. In hepatitis B and C, viral replication is the main cause of liver damage. By reducing the virus's ability to reproduce, these medications help limit liver inflammation and scarring.

- **Hepatitis B:** Drugs like **Tenofovir** and **Entecavir** work by preventing the hepatitis B virus (HBV) from replicating in the liver, thus reducing inflammation and protecting the liver cells from damage. While hepatitis B is not curable, these medications can keep the disease under control.

- **Hepatitis C:** Newer direct-acting antiviral medications such as **Sofosbuvir** combined with other drugs like

189

Ledipasvir or **Velpatasvir** have dramatically improved the outlook for individuals with hepatitis C. These medications work by targeting specific proteins that the virus uses to replicate. Treatment for hepatitis C is now highly effective, with many individuals achieving a sustained viral response, meaning the virus is undetectable in their bloodstream.

2. Anti-Inflammatory Medications

Inflammation is one of the primary causes of liver damage, particularly in non-alcoholic fatty liver disease (NAFLD) and autoimmune liver diseases. Medications that reduce inflammation can help protect the liver from further harm.

- **Corticosteroids** like **Prednisone** may be prescribed in cases of autoimmune hepatitis or cirrhosis to suppress the body's immune response and reduce liver inflammation.

- **Vitamin E** is sometimes used as an antioxidant in patients with NAFLD to reduce oxidative stress and inflammation in the liver. This has been found to be especially helpful in non-diabetic individuals.

3. Diuretics for Cirrhosis

In cases of cirrhosis, one of the complications is the buildup of fluid in the abdomen (ascites). Diuretic medications like **Spironolactone** and **Furosemide** are commonly used to help the body eliminate excess fluid. These medications help prevent the complications of ascites, such as infection, discomfort, and difficulty breathing.

4. Beta-Blockers

For patients with cirrhosis, the blood pressure in the veins leading to the liver can increase, leading to complications like variceal bleeding (bleeding from swollen veins in the esophagus). **Beta-blockers** such as **Propranolol** are used to reduce this pressure and prevent potentially life-threatening bleeding.

Understanding Liver Transplants

A liver transplant is a surgical procedure where a diseased liver is replaced with a healthy liver from a donor. This option is considered when liver function has deteriorated to the point where a person's life is at risk, and there are no other treatment options available.

Who Needs a Liver Transplant?

A liver transplant may be necessary for patients with end-stage liver disease, which can be caused by chronic hepatitis, alcoholic liver disease, autoimmune liver diseases, or cirrhosis. It may also be needed for individuals with liver cancer (though only in certain cases).

Transplantation is a complex process, and not everyone with liver disease is eligible for a transplant. Factors such as the severity of the disease, the overall health of the patient, and the presence of other medical conditions are considered when determining eligibility.

The Process of a Liver Transplant

The transplant process involves multiple stages:

- **Evaluation:** Before a transplant, patients undergo extensive testing to assess the extent of their liver disease and overall health.

- **Donor Match:** A suitable donor liver is necessary for the transplant. A donor liver can come from a living donor (typically a family member) or a deceased donor. The liver must be a match based on blood type, size, and other factors.
- **Surgery:** The transplant surgery itself is a major procedure, where the diseased liver is removed and replaced with the healthy donor liver. The procedure generally takes several hours and requires a hospital stay afterward for recovery.
- **Post-Transplant Care:** After the transplant, patients must take medications to prevent rejection of the new liver. Immunosuppressant drugs are essential to ensure the body accepts the transplant. These medications, while necessary, also come with risks, such as infection.

Risks and Benefits of Liver Transplants

The benefits of liver transplantation are clear: it offers patients a new chance at life. However, the surgery carries risks. These risks include complications like organ rejection, infection, and issues related to the use of immunosuppressant drugs, which can make the body more susceptible to other infections.

The survival rate after a liver transplant has improved dramatically in recent years, but it's important for patients to follow medical advice and maintain a healthy lifestyle to ensure the success of the transplant.

The Risks and Benefits of Medical Interventions

Medical interventions are vital for treating liver disease, but, like all treatments, they come with both risks and benefits. It's important to carefully consider the potential outcomes before proceeding with any treatment option.

Benefits of Medical Treatments

- **Slowing Disease Progression:** Medications and treatments can slow or halt the progression of liver disease, helping prevent further damage. For example, antiviral medications for hepatitis or anti-inflammatory medications for NAFLD can help manage the disease.
- **Symptom Relief:** Many treatments can alleviate symptoms such as pain, swelling, fatigue, and jaundice, improving the quality of life for patients.
- **Life-Saving Interventions:** For individuals with end-stage liver disease or liver cancer, liver transplants provide a life-saving option when all other treatments fail.

Risks of Medical Treatments

- **Side Effects:** Medications, while beneficial, can sometimes cause unwanted side effects. For example, antiviral medications may cause fatigue, gastrointestinal discomfort, or skin rashes. Immunosuppressants used in liver transplants may make patients more prone to infections.
- **Long-Term Complications:** Some treatments, especially medications, may have long-term effects that require careful monitoring by healthcare professionals. For instance, the use of corticosteroids for inflammation may lead to bone thinning or increased risk of diabetes if used for prolonged periods.
- **Organ Rejection in Liver Transplants:** Although liver transplants are often successful, the new liver may be rejected by the body if immune system suppression is not properly managed.

Medical and alternative treatments for liver disease play a critical role in managing and improving liver health. By using a combination of medications, lifestyle changes, and surgical interventions like liver transplants, patients can significantly improve their prognosis and quality of life. However, it is essential to be aware of the potential risks and benefits of each treatment and work closely with healthcare providers to find the best plan of action for each individual.

Exploring Alternative Therapies: A Doctor's Perspective

In today's rapidly evolving world, people are increasingly turning to alternative therapies as a means of supporting their health and well-being. As an experienced medical professional who has spent decades in the field, I can say with certainty that many individuals seeking alternatives to traditional Western medicine are finding these therapies to be valuable, especially when used as complementary tools. However, it's essential to understand that alternative therapies should not replace conventional treatments unless advised by a healthcare provider. Instead, they should be viewed as valuable additions to a holistic approach to health.

What Are Alternative Therapies?

Alternative therapies encompass a broad range of practices that are used instead of standard medical treatments. These therapies may involve different healing practices, such as acupuncture, chiropractic care, homeopathy, naturopathy, and herbal medicine, to name a few. Many of these therapies have been in practice for thousands of years and have a rich history of offering healing and comfort.

While some of these therapies are scientifically backed, others are not fully proven in terms of Western medical standards. Despite the lack of substantial clinical evidence, many people find them helpful for managing chronic conditions, improving overall well-being, and supporting recovery from illness or injury.

As a doctor, I believe in integrating the best of both worlds—the scientifically proven methods of Western medicine, as well as the ancient wisdom and approaches of alternative therapies. It's not about choosing one over the other but about finding a balance that works best for each individual.

Understanding the Benefits

One of the primary reasons alternative therapies have gained so much popularity in recent years is because they often focus on treating the root cause of the problem, not just the symptoms. They emphasize the importance of preventive care, stress reduction, and overall wellness. This holistic approach can sometimes yield better results for people with chronic conditions like digestive disorders, back pain, or stress-related conditions.

Moreover, many alternative therapies have fewer side effects than conventional pharmaceutical treatments. For example, acupuncture and chiropractic care tend to have minimal risks when performed by trained professionals, and many people prefer them for pain management or to address specific health concerns without resorting to medications.

It is also important to note that some of these therapies work best when integrated with a lifestyle change. For example, a person receiving chiropractic care might also benefit from dietary modifications, increased physical activity, and stress management techniques to maximize healing.

Acupuncture, Chiropractic, and Other Therapies

Acupuncture: A Thousand-Year-Old Practice with Modern Relevance

Acupuncture, originating from traditional Chinese medicine, has been practiced for over two millennia. This therapy involves inserting very thin needles into specific points of the body to balance the flow of energy (also known as "qi" or "chi"). Despite its ancient roots, acupuncture has found a firm place in modern healthcare due to its proven effectiveness in treating a variety of ailments.

As a doctor, I have seen acupuncture help patients manage chronic pain, such as back pain, headaches, and even conditions like fibromyalgia. It can also help with digestive problems, stress, and anxiety, and in some cases, it has been shown to boost immune function.

Acupuncture works by stimulating the body's natural healing abilities. Research indicates that the stimulation of certain points on the body triggers the release of endorphins, which are natural painkillers. This can also improve circulation, reduce inflammation, and promote overall relaxation. Acupuncture may be used as a standalone treatment or alongside other medical interventions.

It's important to consult with a licensed acupuncturist or your physician before beginning treatment to ensure it's right for your specific condition.

Chiropractic Care: Aligning the Body's Structure with Its Function

Chiropractic care focuses on diagnosing and treating musculoskeletal disorders, particularly those related to the spine. It is based on the belief that spinal health affects the overall function of the nervous system and the body as a whole. Chiropractors use hands-on spinal manipulation to correct alignment problems, improve posture, and reduce pain.

From my experience, chiropractic care is an effective treatment for musculoskeletal conditions like lower back pain, neck pain, and headaches. In addition to spinal adjustments, chiropractors may also recommend exercises, lifestyle changes, and ergonomic modifications to prevent further injury.

Chiropractic care is often used in conjunction with physical therapy, massage therapy, and other treatments for holistic pain management and overall wellness. The goal is to help patients move better, feel better, and improve their quality of life.

Other Therapies: Homeopathy and Naturopathy

Homeopathy and naturopathy are other alternative therapies that focus on using natural substances and remedies to stimulate the body's healing processes. Homeopathy is based on the principle of "like cures like," where small doses of natural substances that cause symptoms in a healthy person are used to treat similar symptoms in a sick person. While research on homeopathy remains mixed, many individuals report improvements with this gentle approach to healing.

Naturopathy, on the other hand, emphasizes a holistic approach to health, including nutrition, herbal medicine, hydrotherapy, and lifestyle counseling. Naturopathic doctors (NDs) use a variety of treatments to support the body's ability to heal itself, such as recommending specific diets, supplements, and stress management techniques. Both homeopathy and naturopathy work well for people who seek a natural, non-invasive approach to managing chronic illness or improving wellness.

The Role of Supplements and Herbal Medicine

Supplements: Supporting Your Health from the Inside Out

In the world of alternative therapies, supplements play an important role. Many people turn to vitamins, minerals, amino acids, and other dietary supplements to support their health and fill nutritional gaps in their diet. As a professional who has worked with thousands of patients over the years, I can attest to the importance of proper supplementation.

Supplements can offer vital support to the body, especially in cases of deficiencies or specific health concerns. For example, vitamin D supplements are commonly used to support bone health, while omega-3 fatty acids may help reduce inflammation and support heart health.

However, supplements should never replace a balanced diet. The best way to obtain essential nutrients is through a healthy, varied diet, rich in fruits, vegetables, whole grains, and lean proteins. Supplements should be viewed as complementary tools, not as a substitute for proper nutrition.

It's also important to approach supplementation with caution. Not all supplements are created equal, and some may interact with medications or cause adverse reactions. Therefore, it is crucial to consult with a healthcare professional before introducing any new supplements into your routine.

Herbal Medicine: Harnessing Nature's Healing Power

Herbal medicine is one of the oldest forms of medicine and involves using plant-based remedies to treat a wide range of health conditions. For centuries, people across the globe have relied on herbs for their medicinal properties. Modern science has begun to validate many of these traditional remedies, and numerous studies show that herbal medicine can have therapeutic effects on a variety of conditions.

As a practitioner, I have seen the benefits of certain herbs in supporting liver health, reducing inflammation, and improving digestive function. Popular herbs like milk thistle, turmeric, ginger, and dandelion have been extensively studied and shown to provide significant health benefits.

- **Milk Thistle**: Known for its liver-protective properties, milk thistle has been used for centuries to treat liver conditions like cirrhosis and fatty liver disease. Its active compound, silymarin, has antioxidant and anti-inflammatory effects that help to promote liver detoxification and regeneration.

- **Turmeric**: Curcumin, the active compound in turmeric, is a potent anti-inflammatory agent. It is commonly used for joint pain, digestive issues, and liver support. Studies have shown that turmeric may be effective in managing conditions like arthritis, and it may even help protect the liver from damage.

- **Ginger**: Ginger has long been used to treat nausea, digestive issues, and inflammation. It is commonly recommended for people with indigestion, motion sickness, and nausea related to chemotherapy.

While herbal medicine can be incredibly effective, it's crucial to approach it with respect. Herbs are powerful and can interact with medications, especially those used to treat chronic conditions. Always consult with a healthcare provider before using herbal remedies, particularly if you are on prescription medications.

What to Do When Conventional Treatments Aren't Enough

When you're diagnosed with a liver condition, the conventional treatments you're prescribed are typically the first line of defense. These might include medications, lifestyle changes, or in some cases, surgery. However, there comes a time when conventional treatments are no longer enough to keep your liver healthy, especially in chronic conditions like fatty liver disease, cirrhosis, or autoimmune hepatitis. You might feel as though you've reached a dead-end, but don't lose hope – there are still plenty of options to explore.

Reevaluate Your Treatment Plan

If you're not seeing improvement with conventional treatments, the first thing to do is reassess your current plan with your healthcare provider. Sometimes, the medications you're on may not be the right fit for your specific condition. Your doctor might recommend a change in dosage, an alternative drug, or a different treatment altogether. Don't be afraid to ask questions or express concerns about your current regimen.

Lifestyle Modifications

Many liver conditions are exacerbated by poor lifestyle choices, so making changes in your daily routine can make a significant difference. If you haven't already, consider adopting a liver-friendly diet. This might include eating more fruits, vegetables, and whole grains while cutting back on processed foods, sugars, and alcohol. Exercise is equally important; even light activity like walking can improve liver function and reduce the risk of further damage.

If you are overweight or obese, losing even a small amount of weight can help reduce fat buildup in your liver, particularly in the case of non-alcoholic fatty liver disease (NAFLD). Your doctor or dietitian can help you design a personalized weight-loss plan that doesn't compromise your health.

Consider Specialized Care

Sometimes conventional treatments can only do so much, and in these cases, you might need to seek care from a specialist. A hepatologist, a doctor who specializes in liver diseases, can provide more in-depth treatment and help manage complex liver conditions. These specialists have the expertise to explore other treatments and tests that your primary care doctor may not have considered.

Explore Clinical Trials

Another option worth exploring is participation in clinical trials. Clinical trials allow you to access cutting-edge treatments that have not yet been widely released to the public. Your doctor can guide you on how to find legitimate trials and whether you qualify to participate. Though there's no guarantee that the experimental treatment will work, it may offer new hope when conventional options fall short.

Mental and Emotional Health

Dealing with chronic liver disease can be mentally and emotionally taxing. It's important to acknowledge the psychological aspects of illness, which can often be overlooked. Stress and depression can worsen physical symptoms, so addressing mental health should be part of your treatment plan. Seeking therapy, joining support groups, or even talking openly with your doctor about how you feel can provide comfort and boost your mental well-being, which may, in turn, improve your physical health.

Working with Your Doctor to Manage Liver Disease

Managing liver disease requires a strong partnership between you and your healthcare team. The liver is a resilient organ, but it needs constant care to maintain its function, especially when dealing with chronic conditions. Working together with your doctor can help you feel more in control of your health, improve your treatment outcomes, and prevent complications.

Be Honest and Transparent

Open communication with your doctor is essential when managing liver disease. It's important to share everything you know about your lifestyle, including your diet, physical activity level, alcohol consumption, and any over-the-counter or prescription medications you're taking. Sometimes, medications and lifestyle factors can worsen liver disease, so being transparent about these aspects will help your doctor create a treatment plan tailored specifically to your needs.

If you're unsure about something, don't hesitate to ask questions. Your doctor is there to provide guidance and answer any concerns you may have, whether it's about your diagnosis, treatment options, or lifestyle changes. Asking questions also empowers you to become more involved in your care, which can help improve your overall health outcomes.

Understand Your Diagnosis

One of the most important aspects of managing liver disease is fully understanding your diagnosis. Ask your doctor to explain the specifics of your condition, including the stage of the disease, potential complications, and what your prognosis looks like. It's also helpful to know how to monitor your liver health through blood tests, imaging studies, or physical exams. Understanding your liver health on a deeper level will allow you to make informed decisions about your treatment and lifestyle choices.

Follow Your Doctor's Recommendations

Following your doctor's advice is crucial in managing liver disease effectively. This might involve taking prescribed medications regularly, adhering to dietary recommendations, and following up with your doctor for routine checkups. Skipping appointments or neglecting treatment protocols can lead to worsening liver function, so it's essential to stay on track.

If you're prescribed medication, be diligent about taking it as instructed. Some medications can have side effects, so keep track of any changes in your health and report them to your doctor. It may take some time to find the right combination of treatments, but persistence and patience are key to managing your condition.

Work Together to Set Goals

You and your doctor should work together to set realistic and measurable goals for managing your liver disease. These might include things like reducing liver inflammation, achieving a healthy weight, or improving your blood test results. By having clear goals, you can better assess the effectiveness of your treatment plan and make adjustments if necessary. Setting goals also helps you stay motivated and focused on improving your liver health.

Stay Proactive and Be Your Own Advocate

While your doctor plays a critical role in managing your liver disease, you also have a responsibility to take an active role in your own health. This means staying informed, seeking out new treatments when necessary, and advocating for yourself when you feel that your care isn't meeting your needs. If you feel like something isn't working, don't be afraid to get a second opinion or ask for additional tests. Remember that you know your body best, and your doctor should listen to your concerns and collaborate with you to find the most effective treatment.

Integrating Alternative and Conventional Treatments

In recent years, there has been a growing interest in integrating alternative and conventional treatments to manage liver disease. Conventional medicine focuses on evidence-based treatments, like medication and surgery, while alternative treatments include practices such as herbal remedies, acupuncture, and dietary supplements. Combining both approaches can offer more comprehensive care and help manage liver disease more effectively, but it requires careful consideration and a well-coordinated plan with your healthcare provider.

Why Integrate Both Approaches?
Liver disease is complex, and every patient's experience is unique. While conventional treatments are often necessary to address the underlying causes of liver disease, alternative treatments can complement these methods by offering additional ways to improve liver function, reduce symptoms, and promote healing. By combining the best of both worlds, patients may experience faster recovery, improved quality of life, and a better overall outcome.

Herbal Supplements for Liver Health
Several herbal remedies have shown promise in supporting liver health. Milk thistle, dandelion root, turmeric, and artichoke extract are commonly used in alternative medicine for their liver-protective properties. Milk thistle, for instance, contains silymarin, an antioxidant that can help reduce liver inflammation and promote

detoxification. However, it's important to use these remedies under the supervision of your doctor, as they may interact with prescription medications or cause side effects.

Acupuncture and Traditional Chinese Medicine

Acupuncture and other forms of traditional Chinese medicine (TCM) have been used for centuries to treat a variety of health conditions, including liver disease. Acupuncture involves inserting thin needles into specific points on the body to promote healing and balance. Some studies suggest that acupuncture may help reduce liver inflammation and alleviate symptoms like fatigue, which are common in liver disease. If you're considering acupuncture, make sure to find a licensed practitioner who specializes in TCM and consult with your doctor beforehand.

Dietary Interventions and Nutritional Support

A liver-friendly diet is a cornerstone of both conventional and alternative treatments for liver disease. A diet rich in antioxidants, healthy fats, and fiber can reduce inflammation, improve liver function, and promote overall health. Many alternative approaches emphasize whole foods, plant-based diets, and avoiding processed foods, sugars, and alcohol. Your doctor or a nutritionist can guide you on how to incorporate these dietary changes effectively into your treatment plan.

Mind-Body Practices

In addition to physical treatments, mind-body practices like yoga and meditation can help reduce stress, which in turn can improve liver function. Chronic stress can contribute to liver damage, so finding ways to relax and manage stress is crucial. Practices like deep breathing, mindfulness, and gentle exercise can support your liver's healing process and improve your overall well-being.

Consult Your Doctor Before Combining Treatments

Before integrating alternative treatments into your liver disease management plan, it's essential to consult with your doctor. Some alternative remedies can interfere with medications or exacerbate certain conditions. Your doctor will help you evaluate the safety and effectiveness of these treatments based on your individual health needs. It's important to approach alternative treatments with caution, as not all remedies are proven to be safe or effective.

By integrating both alternative and conventional treatments, you can create a well-rounded, personalized plan to manage liver disease. Always remember that the key to successful treatment lies in open communication with your healthcare provider and taking a proactive role in your own care. With the right approach, you can protect and heal your liver, leading to a healthier and more vibrant life.

Chapter 11: Preventing Liver Disease and Maintaining Health

The liver is one of the most essential organs in your body. It's the organ responsible for filtering toxins from your bloodstream, aiding in digestion, storing nutrients, and even helping to regulate your blood sugar levels. Yet, many people neglect liver health until they experience symptoms of a problem. The truth is, preventing liver disease is much more manageable than you might think. By making simple lifestyle changes and adopting healthier habits, you can ensure your liver stays in good shape for years to come. As an experienced doctor in the field, I want to guide you through how to prevent liver disease and maintain a healthy liver.

How to Prevent Fatty Liver and Other Liver Diseases

Fatty liver disease, or hepatic steatosis, is one of the most common liver conditions affecting adults, often due to poor diet, obesity, and a sedentary lifestyle. This condition is progressive, which means it can worsen over time if not addressed properly. However, by understanding how to prevent fatty liver and other liver diseases, you can reduce your risk significantly.

1. **Healthy Diet**
    A well-balanced diet plays a critical role in preventing fatty liver disease. The liver thrives on nutrients found in whole foods like fruits, vegetables, lean proteins, and whole grains. Avoid processed and high-fat foods that contribute to fat buildup in the liver. The Mediterranean diet, rich in fruits, vegetables, nuts, whole grains, and healthy fats like olive oil, is a great example of a

liver-friendly diet.

2. **Control Your Weight**

   Obesity is a leading cause of fatty liver disease. Carrying excess weight, especially around the abdomen, puts a strain on your liver. Losing even a small amount of weight (5-10% of your body weight) can help reduce fat in the liver and improve overall liver function. Maintaining a healthy weight through regular exercise and mindful eating can prevent the onset of fatty liver and other liver-related conditions.

3. **Limit Alcohol Consumption**

   Excessive alcohol consumption is a significant cause of liver disease, particularly cirrhosis. Alcohol can damage liver cells, leading to inflammation and scarring, which can progress to liver failure. While some people can consume alcohol in moderation without issues, it's best to limit alcohol to a safe level or avoid it altogether if you want to protect your liver.

4. **Exercise Regularly**

   Physical activity is a crucial component of liver health. Regular exercise helps to reduce liver fat, lower inflammation, and improve overall metabolism. Aim for at least 150 minutes of moderate-intensity exercise each week, such as walking, swimming, or cycling. Consistency is key; even a daily walk can be incredibly beneficial for your liver.

5. **Avoid Toxins**

   Environmental toxins, including chemicals, pollution, and certain medications, can harm your liver over time. When possible, minimize exposure to harmful substances, including household cleaning products, pesticides, and cigarette smoke. Be sure to follow safety instructions when handling chemicals or taking prescription medications, and always consult your doctor before taking any over-the-counter supplements.

6. **Regular Health Checkups**

Regular medical checkups are essential for identifying liver issues before they become severe. Your doctor can monitor your liver enzymes and other health indicators to ensure that your liver is functioning properly. If you are at risk for liver disease, your doctor may recommend additional tests, such as ultrasounds or biopsies, to detect early signs of liver damage.

Lifestyle Modifications That Keep Your Liver Healthy

Lifestyle choices play a significant role in maintaining the health of your liver. A few simple changes can go a long way in preventing liver disease and ensuring your liver remains in good working order. Here are some key lifestyle modifications to help you protect your liver:

1. **Eat a Liver-Friendly Diet**

Your liver requires the right nutrients to function optimally. Eating a nutrient-dense diet filled with antioxidants, vitamins, and minerals supports liver health. Focus on foods that promote detoxification, such as leafy greens, cruciferous vegetables (like broccoli and cabbage), berries, citrus fruits, and beets. Additionally, foods high in fiber, like whole grains and legumes, help maintain healthy digestion, which reduces the burden on your liver.

2. **Stay Hydrated**

   Drinking plenty of water is essential for liver health. Water helps flush out toxins, supports digestion, and ensures that the liver can filter waste products from the bloodstream. Aim for at least 8 glasses of water a day, and avoid sugary drinks like sodas, which can contribute to fatty liver disease. Herbal teas like dandelion root tea or milk thistle tea may also have liver-supportive properties, but they should be used with caution and under the guidance of a healthcare professional.

3. **Exercise Regularly**

   Exercise not only helps manage your weight but also improves liver function by promoting better circulation and fat metabolism. Regular physical activity helps reduce fat buildup in the liver and lowers the risk of developing conditions like non-alcoholic fatty liver disease (NAFLD) and cirrhosis. Aim for at least 30 minutes of moderate exercise on most days of the week. Simple activities like walking, jogging, or cycling can make a significant difference.

4. **Quit Smoking**

   Smoking is one of the most harmful habits for your liver. The chemicals in tobacco smoke can harm liver cells, promote inflammation, and contribute to conditions like liver cancer. If you smoke, quitting is one of the best things you can do for your liver and overall health. If you're struggling to quit, seek support from a healthcare professional or smoking cessation program to help you succeed.

5. **Limit Alcohol Consumption**

   While a glass of wine or a beer now and then may not

cause harm, excessive alcohol consumption is a leading cause of liver damage. Chronic alcohol use can lead to fatty liver, cirrhosis, and even liver cancer. It's important to understand your limits and follow recommended guidelines for alcohol consumption. If you're concerned about your drinking habits, it's best to speak with a healthcare provider for advice and guidance.

6. **Manage Stress**

Chronic stress can negatively affect your liver. Stress hormones, such as cortisol, can contribute to inflammation and other health issues. Finding ways to manage stress, such as through mindfulness, meditation, yoga, or deep breathing exercises, can help keep your liver in good condition. A relaxed mind leads to a relaxed body, which is crucial for liver health.

7. **Get Enough Sleep**

Quality sleep is essential for overall health and well-being. During sleep, your body repairs and regenerates itself, including the liver. Poor sleep patterns, on the other hand, can contribute to liver dysfunction and other health issues. Aim for 7-9 hours of sleep per night to allow your liver to recover and function optimally.

8. **Avoid Overuse of Medications**

Certain medications, including over-the-counter painkillers like acetaminophen (Tylenol), can put strain on your liver if taken in excess. Always follow the dosage instructions carefully and consult your doctor before using any new medications, especially if you have a history of liver disease. If you need to take prescription medications regularly, your doctor may monitor your liver function with blood tests.

Regular Screenings and Liver Health Tests

Even if you're following a healthy lifestyle, it's still important to monitor the health of your liver with regular screenings and tests. Early detection of liver disease can help prevent further complications and improve the effectiveness of treatments. Here's what you need to know about liver health tests and screenings:

1. **Blood Tests**
    One of the most common ways to assess liver function is through blood tests that measure liver enzymes, proteins, and other substances produced by the liver. Elevated liver enzymes (AST, ALT, ALP, and bilirubin) can indicate liver damage or inflammation. Regular blood tests can help detect issues early, allowing for timely intervention.

2. **Ultrasound**
    Ultrasound is a non-invasive imaging technique that can help assess liver health. It can identify fatty liver, cirrhosis, liver tumors, and other abnormalities. If you're at risk for liver disease due to factors like obesity or a family history of liver issues, an ultrasound may be recommended as part of your routine checkup.

3. **CT Scans and MRIs**
    In some cases, a doctor may recommend a CT scan or MRI to get a more detailed image of the liver. These imaging tests are particularly useful for detecting liver tumors, cysts, and other structural abnormalities that might not be visible through an ultrasound.

4. **Liver Biopsy**

   A liver biopsy is a procedure in which a small sample of liver tissue is removed and examined under a microscope. While this test is not commonly done, it can help confirm the presence of liver diseases such as cirrhosis, hepatitis, or non-alcoholic fatty liver disease (NAFLD). This test is typically reserved for cases where other tests have not provided a definitive diagnosis.

5. **FibroScan**

   A newer test, FibroScan, is a non-invasive procedure that measures liver stiffness. This can help determine the level of fibrosis (scarring) in the liver, which is an indicator of liver damage. It's particularly useful for assessing the progression of liver diseases like cirrhosis or fatty liver.

6. **Liver Function Test**

   This test measures the level of various substances in the blood to assess how well the liver is functioning. These tests measure proteins, enzymes, and bilirubin levels to check the liver's ability to produce proteins, break down waste products, and metabolize drugs.

The Importance of Regular Monitoring and Blood Work

As a physician with decades of experience, I've seen countless patients whose liver issues could have been identified and addressed sooner if they had simply been more aware of the importance of regular monitoring and blood work. The liver, while often an unsung hero in the body, plays a pivotal role in almost every process that keeps us alive and well. It detoxifies the blood, produces proteins essential for blood clotting, stores glycogen for energy, and plays a central role in digestion. Given all that the liver does, ensuring its health should be a top priority in maintaining overall wellness.

Understanding the Importance of Regular Monitoring

Liver disease, in many cases, develops slowly, without noticeable symptoms, and can become quite severe by the time signs become evident. This is why early detection through regular monitoring is crucial. By undergoing routine blood tests, you're essentially catching potential liver issues before they have a chance to progress into something more serious, such as fatty liver disease, cirrhosis, or even liver cancer.

Why Regular Monitoring is Essential

1. **Silent Progression of Liver Disease** Many liver conditions, like non-alcoholic fatty liver disease (NAFLD), progress silently over time without any obvious signs. It's easy to feel fine and assume all is well, but liver damage can be taking place at a microscopic level. Regular check-ups allow for blood tests that can detect early signs of liver stress, such as elevated liver enzymes or other markers that indicate an issue.

2. **Early Detection of Liver Disease** The sooner liver damage is detected, the more likely it is that appropriate steps can be taken to reverse or at least halt its progression. For example, elevated liver enzymes can be an early indication of inflammation or damage to liver cells. If these are detected early, dietary and lifestyle changes can be implemented to improve liver health, potentially preventing

further damage and more severe conditions down the road.

3. **Identifying Risk Factors Early** Regular blood tests can help identify risk factors for liver disease, such as high cholesterol, high blood sugar, or elevated blood pressure. These conditions are often linked to fatty liver disease and can increase your risk of liver-related complications. By identifying these risk factors early, you can take action to manage them, thus reducing the potential for liver damage in the future.

4. **Baseline Liver Health Tracking** Blood tests provide valuable baseline data about your liver's function and health. With these markers in hand, your healthcare provider can track changes over time and quickly identify any deterioration in liver function. This is particularly important for individuals with known liver conditions or those who are at high risk due to factors like obesity, diabetes, or excessive alcohol use.

5. **Monitoring Medication Impact** Many medications can affect liver function. Whether it's over-the-counter pain relievers, prescription drugs, or even certain herbal supplements, some medications can put strain on the liver. Regular blood work is essential to ensure that your medications are not harming your liver, especially if you have pre-existing liver conditions.

How Blood Tests Help

Blood tests are the primary tool used to monitor liver health. These tests measure various biomarkers that give an indication of how well the liver is functioning. The most commonly tested biomarkers include liver enzymes, bilirubin levels, and albumin levels. These tests help to provide insight into the health of the liver and whether it's processing substances like toxins, waste, and nutrients efficiently.

Key tests include:

- **Liver Function Tests (LFTs):** This panel measures several enzymes like AST, ALT, ALP, and GGT, which are indicators of liver health.
- **Complete Blood Count (CBC):** This test can help assess the overall health of your liver by measuring the number of red blood cells, white blood cells, and platelets in your blood.
- **Bilirubin Test:** Bilirubin is a substance produced by the liver when red blood cells break down. If bilirubin levels are elevated, it could indicate a liver problem.
- **Prothrombin Time (PT):** This test measures how long it takes for blood to clot, which can be affected by liver health.

By regularly monitoring these markers, any changes can be detected early, providing the opportunity to make lifestyle modifications or seek further treatment if necessary.

How to Track Your Liver Health Over Time

Liver health is something that can be maintained, improved, or sometimes reversed through thoughtful and consistent monitoring. However, this requires an understanding of how to track liver health over time and when to seek professional guidance.

1. Know Your Baseline Liver Health

Tracking your liver health begins with establishing a baseline. This means understanding your liver function at the point when you are feeling healthy and symptom-free. For those without pre-existing liver conditions, this could simply be done through annual check-ups.

A baseline liver function test will provide data on the normal levels of liver enzymes, bilirubin, and other relevant markers. These values will become your reference point for future testing, allowing for comparisons as time goes on. If you already have a liver condition, your baseline might be slightly altered, but it still provides valuable insight into how your liver is functioning at the start of your journey.

2. Regular Blood Tests

Once you have a baseline, it's important to schedule regular follow-up blood tests to monitor any changes. For those with liver disease, the frequency of testing might be higher (e.g., quarterly or semi-annually). These tests should measure the same markers as the baseline to track any improvements or deterioration.

In between testing, you can observe for physical symptoms that could indicate a change in liver function, such as:

- Yellowing of the skin or eyes (jaundice)
- Unexplained weight loss or fatigue
- Abdominal pain or swelling
- Dark urine or pale stools
- Skin rashes or changes

If you notice any of these signs, it's critical to follow up with a healthcare provider promptly.

3. Lifestyle and Dietary Tracking

Another vital aspect of tracking liver health involves lifestyle factors such as diet, exercise, and alcohol consumption. Keeping a food and drink diary can help you notice patterns that may negatively impact your liver, such as excessive intake of fatty foods, alcohol, or processed sugars. By maintaining a balanced diet with nutrient-rich foods, such as vegetables, fruits, and lean proteins, and reducing or eliminating alcohol intake, you can actively promote liver health.

Physical activity is equally important in maintaining a healthy liver. Regular exercise helps reduce body fat, a common cause of fatty liver disease. Keep track of your physical activity levels, ensuring that you're engaging in at least 150 minutes of moderate-intensity exercise per week.

4. Monitor Symptoms and Side Effects

Tracking your symptoms and side effects can also provide valuable information. Some people with liver disease don't experience symptoms until the damage is quite advanced. Keeping a journal of any changes in your energy levels, digestion, skin, and weight can help detect early signs of liver dysfunction.

5. Consult with Your Doctor Regularly

In addition to at-home tracking, it's vital to consult with your healthcare provider regularly. They can order blood tests, imaging studies, or biopsies to help track the progression of any liver disease you may have. They can also adjust your treatment plan based on the results of these tests to help manage or reverse liver damage.

What Your Liver Enzyme Levels Mean

Your liver enzymes play a crucial role in your liver's function, as they help break down food and toxins in the body. Monitoring your liver enzyme levels provides valuable insight into your liver's health. These enzymes are proteins produced by the liver that are released into the bloodstream when liver cells are damaged. Elevated levels of liver enzymes can indicate liver inflammation, injury, or disease.

1. Aspartate Aminotransferase (AST) and Alanine Aminotransferase (ALT)

AST and ALT are two of the most commonly tested liver enzymes. Both are found in liver cells, and when the liver is damaged, these enzymes leak into the bloodstream. Elevated levels of AST and ALT typically signal liver injury, though it's important to note that these enzymes can also be elevated in non-liver-related conditions, such as muscle injury or heart disease. However, significantly high levels may indicate liver disease, such as hepatitis, fatty liver disease, or cirrhosis.

2. Gamma-Glutamyl Transferase (GGT)

GGT is another liver enzyme commonly tested in liver function panels. It helps in the metabolism of certain toxins. Elevated GGT levels can indicate liver disease, especially alcohol-related liver damage, bile duct issues, or other liver conditions. However, this enzyme can also be elevated in other conditions like heart disease or pancreatitis.

3. Alkaline Phosphatase (ALP)

ALP is an enzyme that helps break down proteins. It's present in several tissues throughout the body, including the liver, bones, and kidneys. High levels of ALP can indicate liver disease, especially those affecting the bile ducts or liver tumors.

4. Bilirubin

Bilirubin is a substance produced by the liver during the breakdown of red blood cells. Elevated bilirubin levels in the blood can cause jaundice, which is a yellowing of the skin and eyes. High bilirubin levels can indicate liver conditions, such as hepatitis or cirrhosis, or issues with bile flow in the liver.

5. Albumin and Prothrombin Time (PT)

Albumin is a protein produced by the liver that helps maintain blood volume and pressure. Low albumin levels can indicate liver dysfunction. Prothrombin time measures how long it takes for blood to clot and is used to evaluate liver function. An elevated PT can indicate liver damage or disease, as the liver produces proteins involved in blood clotting.

Building a Liver-Healthy Future

Your liver is a remarkable organ. It works tirelessly every single day to detoxify your body, produce bile to help digest food, store vitamins and minerals, and even help regulate your hormones. It is essential for your overall health and well-being, yet often, we neglect it until something goes wrong. The good news is, with some mindful care and small, consistent adjustments, you can build a liver-healthy future that supports you for years to come.

To understand the importance of liver health, let's first take a moment to appreciate the crucial role your liver plays in your body. It processes everything you consume—food, drinks, medications, and even toxins in the environment. It also helps with the regulation of fat storage, blood sugar levels, and cholesterol balance. It's one of the few organs that can regenerate itself, but this process isn't infinite. Over time, if we don't take care of it, the liver can become overburdened, leading to conditions such as fatty liver disease, cirrhosis, or even liver cancer.

Building a liver-healthy future starts with **prevention** and **mindful living**. It requires consistency, knowledge, and the commitment to making lasting changes that support liver function. By developing healthy habits today, you can avoid the dangerous consequences of poor liver health and keep your liver strong and efficient well into the future.

1. Understanding Your Liver's Role

The liver is truly one of the hardest-working organs in your body. It plays a key role in digestion by producing bile, which helps break down fats in your food. It also filters harmful substances from your bloodstream, including alcohol, drugs, and environmental toxins. But did you know that the liver also contributes to hormone regulation, blood sugar control, and the synthesis of proteins essential for blood clotting?

The liver's multitasking nature means that if it gets overwhelmed, it can no longer perform these tasks properly, leading to a cascade of health problems. That's why building a liver-healthy future starts with a deeper understanding of this organ's role in your daily life. When you realize how much it supports your health, you'll have the motivation to care for it better.

2. Key Factors that Support Liver Health

Several factors are vital for maintaining the health and function of your liver. Here are some of the key elements that contribute to a healthy liver and that you should consider integrating into your lifestyle:

- **Healthy Diet**: The foods you eat play a critical role in supporting liver function. A balanced diet, rich in fruits, vegetables, lean proteins, and healthy fats, can reduce the burden on your liver. Specific foods, such as leafy greens, garlic, turmeric, and cruciferous vegetables like broccoli, are especially beneficial for liver health. They help reduce inflammation and support the liver's detoxification processes.

- **Regular Exercise**: Physical activity promotes good blood circulation and helps maintain a healthy weight. Regular exercise can prevent fatty liver disease, which is closely linked to obesity and metabolic conditions like diabetes. Exercise also aids in regulating blood sugar and cholesterol, two key factors that impact liver health.

- **Hydration**: Drinking enough water is essential for your liver to flush out toxins. Dehydration can slow down the detoxification process, which places additional stress on the liver. Aim to drink at least 8 glasses of water a day, and avoid excessive consumption of sugary drinks or alcohol.

- **Moderating Alcohol Intake**: Chronic alcohol consumption is one of the primary causes of liver disease. If you drink, do so in moderation. Women should limit alcohol to one drink per day, and men should limit it to two. If you are at risk for liver disease, or if you have been diagnosed with fatty liver or cirrhosis, it may be best to avoid alcohol completely.

- **Avoiding Toxins**: Environmental toxins, such as pesticides, chemicals in cleaning products, and pollutants, can put additional strain on your liver. Use natural products when possible, and make sure to protect yourself from chemicals by wearing gloves and masks when handling them.

3. Recognizing Early Warning Signs

In many cases, liver disease doesn't show symptoms until it has progressed to a more severe stage. However, there are some early warning signs that you can look out for. These include:

- Unexplained fatigue
- Jaundice (yellowing of the skin or eyes)
- Abdominal pain or discomfort, particularly in the upper right side
- Dark urine and pale stools
- Swelling in the legs or abdomen (ascites)
- Nausea or vomiting after eating

If you notice any of these symptoms, it's important to seek medical advice and get your liver function tested. Early intervention is crucial for preventing further damage and ensuring a healthy liver.

4. Lifelong Commitment to Liver Health

Building a liver-healthy future isn't something that happens overnight. It's a lifelong commitment to making choices that support liver health. Here are some steps you can take to ensure your liver stays in peak condition:

- **Annual Liver Check-Ups**: Regular check-ups with your doctor are essential for monitoring liver health, especially if you are at risk for liver disease due to factors like obesity, diabetes, or a family history of liver conditions.

- **Avoid Self-Medicating**: Some over-the-counter medications and supplements can be harmful to your liver when taken in excess or for extended periods. Always consult your doctor before taking new medications or supplements.

- **Stay Informed**: Stay up to date with the latest research on liver health. Science is always evolving, and new breakthroughs in liver care may offer better ways to prevent or treat liver disease.

Building a liver-healthy future requires awareness, commitment, and effort, but it is completely possible. By taking action now, you can prevent liver disease and ensure a strong, vibrant liver for years to come.

Setting Long-Term Goals for Liver Health

When it comes to liver health, one of the most powerful tools you have is **goal setting**. Setting long-term goals for liver health not only gives you direction but also provides you with the motivation to stick with your healthy habits. It helps to frame liver care as an ongoing journey, rather than a one-time event.

1. Why Setting Long-Term Goals is Important

Your liver is a vital organ that affects your overall well-being. From its role in digestion and detoxification to hormone regulation and fat metabolism, it has a hand in nearly every bodily process. For this reason, you should treat liver health as a long-term investment.

Setting goals helps you stay focused on making decisions that support your liver, such as improving your diet, exercising regularly, and reducing alcohol intake. It also empowers you to take charge of your health in a more proactive and sustainable way. Instead of waiting for liver problems to occur, you are working to prevent them.

2. Steps to Setting Effective Liver Health Goals

The key to setting effective long-term goals for liver health is to be specific, measurable, and realistic. Here's how you can get started:

- **Evaluate Your Current Liver Health**: The first step in setting any goal is to assess where you currently stand. Are you at risk for liver disease? Do you have any symptoms or a family history of liver issues? A liver function test and a consultation with your doctor can help you get a clearer picture of your current health.

- **Establish Clear Goals**: Once you have an understanding of where you are, you can set clear, achievable goals. For example, your goals could be to lose 10 pounds over the next three months, cut down on alcohol consumption, or add more liver-healthy foods to your diet. Make sure your goals are specific, measurable, and realistic for your lifestyle.

- **Set Short-Term and Long-Term Goals**: Short-term goals could include things like exercising three times a week or drinking more water daily. Long-term goals could involve more significant changes, such as achieving a healthy body weight or reversing early signs of fatty liver disease. Both types of goals are important in maintaining liver health.

- **Track Progress**: Set up a system to monitor your progress. You might keep a health journal or use an app to track your diet, exercise, and any symptoms you may have. Regularly checking in on your goals helps you stay accountable and make adjustments when necessary.

- **Stay Adaptable**: Life can throw challenges your way, and there may be times when you need to adjust your goals. If your progress slows down, don't get discouraged—adjust your plan and keep moving forward. Remember, building a healthy liver is a long-term commitment.

3. Long-Term Benefits of Healthy Liver Goals

When you focus on long-term goals for liver health, you not only improve the function of this vital organ but also benefit your overall health. Here are some of the long-term benefits of committing to liver health:

- **Improved Digestion and Detoxification**: A healthy liver processes toxins more effectively, reducing the burden on other organs, like the kidneys and digestive system. This can lead to better energy, improved digestion, and overall vitality.

- **Preventing Liver Disease**: Taking care of your liver by following a healthy lifestyle can prevent conditions like fatty liver disease, cirrhosis, and liver cancer. Prevention is always more effective than treatment, so early interventions can safeguard you against more serious health issues down the road.

- **Better Mental Clarity**: Since the liver plays a role in hormone balance and detoxification, a healthier liver can lead to clearer thinking, improved mood, and better sleep.

By setting long-term goals and taking proactive steps, you create a future where liver health is a priority and a reality. Regular check-ups, lifestyle adjustments, and healthy habits will allow you to thrive for years to come.

Creating a Personal Action Plan for Ongoing Liver Support

Once you've set your long-term goals for liver health, it's time to **create a personal action plan**. An action plan provides you with the structure and tools you need to stay on track and make progress. It is a roadmap for incorporating liver-healthy habits into your daily life.

1. Assess Your Current Lifestyle

Before creating an action plan, it's important to evaluate your current lifestyle. This includes your diet, exercise routine, stress levels, alcohol consumption, and any other factors that could impact liver health. Identifying areas for improvement will help you prioritize your goals.

2. Make Small, Sustainable Changes

Rather than trying to change everything at once, focus on making small, sustainable changes. Here are a few areas to focus on:

- **Diet**: Focus on adding more liver-friendly foods to your diet, such as leafy greens, fatty fish, garlic, turmeric, and cruciferous vegetables. Reduce processed foods, sugar, and unhealthy fats.

- **Exercise**: Incorporate more physical activity into your routine. Aim for at least 150 minutes of moderate exercise each week, which can include walking, swimming, or cycling.

- **Hydration**: Drink plenty of water throughout the day. Staying hydrated supports your liver's detoxification processes and ensures your body functions optimally.

- **Alcohol Consumption**: If you drink alcohol, make sure to do so in moderation. Consider having alcohol-free days each week to give your liver time to recover.

3. Create a Routine

Consistency is key when it comes to liver health. Create a daily routine that supports your goals. For example, you could start each morning with a glass of warm lemon water to support liver detox, incorporate healthy meals into your week, and schedule time for regular exercise.

4. Regular Monitoring and Adjustments

Track your progress regularly and adjust your plan as necessary. If you feel like you're not making progress, take a step back and evaluate what might be holding you back. Are you staying consistent with your diet and exercise? Are there any external factors—like stress or environmental toxins—that you need to address?

5. Seek Professional Guidance

Incorporating professional advice into your action plan is invaluable. Regular check-ups with your healthcare provider are essential to track liver function and receive expert guidance. They can also help you adjust your plan based on your personal health needs.

By creating and following a personal action plan for ongoing liver support, you ensure that your liver health remains a priority. The key is consistency and patience—your liver will thank you for the effort.

Conclusion

As you come to the end of this book, I want you to feel empowered with a new perspective on liver health. Think of this moment as the beginning of a healthier you, a new chapter where you take charge of your liver's well-being. Your liver plays a pivotal role in your body's overall health and vitality. Every decision you make from here on out—what you eat, how active you are, the choices you make for your lifestyle—will contribute to how well your liver functions.

The liver's ability to regenerate is extraordinary, but it relies on you to give it the right tools. By understanding the role of the liver and how to protect it, you've already taken an important step towards a healthier future. A damaged liver doesn't have to be permanent. With the right diet, exercise, stress management, and detox practices, you can support your liver in its natural healing process. Don't forget, every small change you make to improve your health adds up over time.

Remember, it's never too late to start. No matter your age or current health condition, focusing on liver health can help prevent serious diseases and improve your quality of life. If you've been struggling with fatigue, weight gain, or inflammation, know that these could be signs of liver distress that you now have the tools to address. It's time for a new beginning, a fresh start that will pave the way for lasting liver health.

Empowering Yourself with Knowledge and Action

Knowledge is power, and by now, you should feel armed with a wealth of understanding about the liver, its functions, and how to protect it. But knowledge alone is not enough. To truly make a difference, you must act. The tips, remedies, and lifestyle changes outlined in this book are not just suggestions; they are proven strategies that can transform your liver health and overall well-being.

Empowering yourself starts with taking the first step. Perhaps you'll begin by eliminating processed foods from your diet or incorporating liver-friendly foods like leafy greens and antioxidant-rich fruits into your meals. It's all about making conscious decisions that serve your liver, and by extension, your entire body. Take the time to research more on the subject, engage with health professionals, and stay up-to-date with the latest scientific advancements. Your liver is your ally in maintaining good health, and treating it with respect can lead to a more energetic, vibrant life.

Action doesn't require perfection. Small, consistent changes will have a lasting impact. Set achievable goals like drinking more water daily, getting regular exercise, or incorporating liver-supporting herbs into your routine. As you take action, keep track of your progress, and celebrate each victory—no matter how small. As your liver heals and your body responds positively, you'll see the powerful connection between your actions and your health.

Don't wait for a health crisis to motivate you. You are in control, and your liver will thank you for the care and attention you provide today and in the future. Knowledge and action together form the foundation of a liver-healthy life.

Final Tips for a Healthy Liver and a Vital Life

Now that you have a deeper understanding of liver health, it's important to remember that maintaining a healthy liver is a lifelong commitment. A vital life doesn't just happen overnight—it's the result of consistent effort and mindful choices. As we conclude this book, I want to leave you with some final tips that will help ensure your liver remains strong and capable for years to come.

First, make liver health a daily priority. This doesn't mean obsessing over every meal or workout, but it does mean incorporating liver-friendly habits into your routine. A balanced diet rich in vegetables, healthy fats, and lean proteins will provide your liver with the nutrients it needs to function efficiently. Incorporating anti-inflammatory foods, such as turmeric and ginger, can also offer additional protection against liver stress.

Second, manage stress. Chronic stress can take a toll on your liver, as well as your overall well-being. Incorporate relaxation techniques into your life, such as deep breathing, meditation, or simple walks in nature. These activities not only help calm your mind but also provide the liver with the opportunity to heal and regenerate.

Third, don't neglect exercise. Regular physical activity helps the liver in its detoxification process, improves circulation, and boosts your metabolism. Aim for at least 30 minutes of moderate exercise most days of the week. This can include walking, swimming, or yoga—whatever works best for you.

Finally, avoid excessive alcohol consumption, limit exposure to toxins, and be cautious with medications. These simple yet powerful actions can significantly reduce the burden on your liver, helping it maintain its crucial functions.

Taking care of your liver is taking care of your future. By following these tips and maintaining a holistic approach to health, you are setting the stage for a long, healthy, and vital life. Keep your liver in the best possible condition, and it will serve you well for years to come.

Appendices

Liver Health Resources and References

Your liver is the body's primary organ for detoxification and a central hub in maintaining overall well-being. Keeping it in optimal condition is essential for a long, healthy life. Fortunately, many reliable resources are available to help you support your liver's health, stay informed, and make the best choices for your well-being.

Books on Liver Health

Several well-respected authors and experts have written extensively about the liver, its function, and how to keep it healthy. Here are a few key books you should consider reading for a deeper understanding:

- **"The Liver Cure" by Dr. Russell Blaylock**
  Dr. Blaylock's book is a comprehensive guide to liver health, providing natural solutions to liver diseases, including fatty liver disease, cirrhosis, and hepatitis. His focus is on how diet, lifestyle changes, and certain supplements can support liver function.

- **"The Liver Detox Diet" by Dr. Jeffrey L. Shapiro**
  Dr. Shapiro offers a guide to cleansing the liver through diet. This book explains how food choices impact liver function and provides practical tips for detoxing and improving liver health through nutrition.

- **"Liver Healing Diet" by Michelle B. Rozen**
  This book provides readers with a liver-healthy diet plan,

offering tips on how to avoid common foods that harm the liver, while also presenting recipes to support liver detoxification.

Websites and Online Resources

The internet is filled with valuable information that can assist you in learning more about liver health and well-being. Here are some reliable websites to explore:

- **American Liver Foundation (www.liverfoundation.org):** A trusted source of information on liver diseases, the American Liver Foundation provides resources for patients, healthcare providers, and the general public. It also offers advocacy, education, and community support for those affected by liver diseases.

- **Mayo Clinic (www.mayoclinic.org):** Mayo Clinic provides extensive resources on liver conditions, such as fatty liver disease, cirrhosis, hepatitis, and liver cancer. It also offers tips on liver care, diet, and exercise.

- **National Institute of Diabetes and Digestive and Kidney Diseases (www.niddk.nih.gov):** This branch of the National Institutes of Health (NIH) offers research-based information on a range of liver diseases, including guidelines for treatment, diagnosis, and prevention.

- **Liver Health Connection (www.liverhealthconnection.com):** A non-profit organization dedicated to providing liver health education, this site features in-depth articles on liver diseases, liver-friendly recipes, lifestyle tips, and more.

Professional Organizations

For ongoing support and updated information, you may want to connect with the following professional organizations:

- **The American Association for the Study of Liver Diseases (AASLD):**
  This professional organization is dedicated to advancing research, education, and practice in liver disease. They host conferences, provide guidelines, and publish the Journal of Hepatology, a well-regarded resource for healthcare professionals.

- **The Hepatitis B Foundation:**
  This non-profit organization is focused on raising awareness about hepatitis B, its prevention, and treatment options. It offers resources for both patients and healthcare providers.

- **The World Hepatitis Alliance:**
  A global organization that advocates for people affected by viral hepatitis. It offers educational tools, events, and a directory of global resources for liver health.

Appendix 2: Liver-Friendly Recipes and Meal Plans

Maintaining a liver-friendly diet is a powerful way to support your liver's health. A balanced, whole-food diet that minimizes processed foods, unhealthy fats, and sugars can reduce the burden on your liver and improve its function. Below are some liver-friendly recipes and meal plans that can be incorporated into your diet.

Liver-Friendly Recipes

1. Healthy Avocado Salad

Ingredients:

- 1 ripe avocado, diced
- 1 cup cherry tomatoes, halved
- ½ cucumber, sliced
- 1 tablespoon olive oil
- 1 tablespoon fresh lemon juice
- Salt and pepper, to taste
- Fresh herbs (parsley or cilantro)

Instructions:

1. Combine the diced avocado, tomatoes, and cucumber in a bowl.
2. Drizzle with olive oil and lemon juice.
3. Season with salt and pepper, then toss gently.
4. Garnish with fresh herbs for extra flavor and nutrients.

Why it's good for your liver:
Avocados are rich in healthy fats that support liver detoxification and help reduce inflammation. Olive oil is also beneficial for reducing liver fat and improving liver enzyme levels.

2. Grilled Salmon with Quinoa and Spinach

Ingredients:

- 2 salmon fillets
- 1 cup quinoa
- 2 cups fresh spinach
- 1 tablespoon olive oil
- Lemon wedges
- Salt and pepper, to taste
- Fresh dill or parsley

Instructions:

1. Rinse the quinoa under cold water and cook according to package instructions.
2. Heat a grill pan and brush with olive oil. Grill the salmon fillets for about 3-4 minutes per side until fully cooked.
3. Sauté the spinach in olive oil until wilted.
4. Serve the grilled salmon over quinoa with sautéed spinach on the side.
5. Garnish with fresh dill or parsley and a squeeze of lemon juice.

Why it's good for your liver:

Salmon is rich in omega-3 fatty acids, which help reduce inflammation and promote liver health. Quinoa is a whole grain that provides fiber and nutrients that support detoxification.

3. Turmeric-Ginger Smoothie

Ingredients:

- 1 cup unsweetened almond milk
- 1 teaspoon ground turmeric
- 1 teaspoon fresh ginger, grated
- 1 banana
- 1 tablespoon honey (optional)

- Ice cubes (optional)

Instructions:

1. Add almond milk, turmeric, ginger, banana, and honey into a blender.
2. Blend until smooth, adding ice cubes if you prefer a colder drink.
3. Pour into a glass and enjoy.

Why it's good for your liver:

Turmeric and ginger are known for their anti-inflammatory properties, which help protect the liver from oxidative damage and support detoxification.

Liver-Friendly Meal Plan

Day 1:

- **Breakfast:** Oatmeal topped with chia seeds, blueberries, and a drizzle of honey.
- **Lunch:** Grilled chicken with a side of steamed broccoli and quinoa.
- **Snack:** Carrot sticks with hummus.
- **Dinner:** Baked cod with roasted sweet potatoes and sautéed spinach.

Day 2:

- **Breakfast:** Smoothie with spinach, banana, chia seeds, and almond milk.
- **Lunch:** Quinoa salad with mixed greens, chickpeas, and olive oil dressing.
- **Snack:** Apple slices with almond butter.

- **Dinner:** Grilled salmon with asparagus and wild rice.

Day 3:

- **Breakfast:** Scrambled eggs with spinach and tomatoes.
- **Lunch:** Turkey and avocado lettuce wraps with cucumber and tomato salad.
- **Snack:** Mixed berries and a handful of almonds.
- **Dinner:** Stir-fry with tofu, bell peppers, broccoli, and brown rice.

This meal plan focuses on nutrient-dense foods that promote liver health, reduce inflammation, and prevent oxidative stress.

Appendix 3: Glossary of Key Terms

Understanding the terminology related to liver health is essential for better comprehension of the subject matter. Below is a glossary of important terms to help you navigate your journey toward better liver health.

1. Cirrhosis

A chronic liver disease marked by irreversible scarring of liver tissue. It is often caused by excessive alcohol consumption, viral hepatitis, or fatty liver disease.

2. Fatty Liver Disease (NAFLD/NASH)

A condition in which excess fat builds up in the liver, potentially leading to inflammation and liver damage. Non-Alcoholic Fatty Liver Disease (NAFLD) and Non-Alcoholic Steatohepatitis (NASH) are the most common types.

3. Hepatitis

Inflammation of the liver, typically caused by a viral infection. Hepatitis A, B, and C are the most common forms.

4. Liver Enzymes

Proteins produced by the liver that help with various biochemical processes. Elevated liver enzymes can indicate liver damage or disease.

5. Detoxification

The process by which the liver breaks down toxins, waste products, and harmful substances from the body. Supporting liver detoxification is key to maintaining liver health.

6. Antioxidants

Molecules that protect cells from oxidative stress and free radical damage. They are essential for liver health and can be found in various fruits, vegetables, and supplements.

7. Jaundice

A condition characterized by yellowing of the skin and eyes, often caused by liver dysfunction or damage.

8. Fibrosis

The formation of scar tissue in the liver as a result of ongoing liver injury. Fibrosis can progress to cirrhosis if untreated.

9. Bile

A digestive fluid produced by the liver that helps break down fats and absorb fat-soluble vitamins in the digestive tract.

10. Steatosis

The accumulation of fat in liver cells. This condition can be a precursor to fatty liver disease if not addressed.

Frequently Asked Questions (FAQ)

1. What is liver disease, and how does it affect the body?

Liver disease refers to any condition that impairs the liver's ability to function properly. The liver is responsible for many essential tasks such as detoxifying the blood, producing bile for digestion, storing nutrients, and regulating blood sugar levels. When the liver is damaged, it can no longer perform these functions as efficiently, leading to a buildup of toxins in the body, digestive problems, and other severe health complications. Common liver diseases include fatty liver disease, cirrhosis, hepatitis, and liver cancer.

2. What are the symptoms of liver disease?

The symptoms of liver disease can vary depending on the severity and type of liver condition. Some common signs to watch for include:

- Fatigue or feeling unusually tired
- Jaundice (yellowing of the skin or eyes)
- Abdominal pain, especially in the upper right side
- Dark urine
- Pale or clay-colored stools
- Swelling in the abdomen or legs
- Nausea or vomiting

- Unexplained weight loss
- Itchy skin

It's important to note that liver disease often doesn't show symptoms until it has reached an advanced stage. This is why regular check-ups are important to detect liver issues early.

3. What are the main causes of liver disease?

Liver disease can result from a variety of factors. Some of the most common causes include:

- **Alcohol Abuse**: Excessive drinking can cause liver inflammation, leading to fatty liver, cirrhosis, and other liver diseases.
- **Hepatitis B and C**: These viral infections can cause severe liver damage if left untreated. They are commonly spread through blood or bodily fluids.
- **Non-Alcoholic Fatty Liver Disease (NAFLD)**: This condition is often associated with obesity, diabetes, high cholesterol, and poor diet, leading to fat buildup in the liver.
- **Medications and Toxins**: Some medications, when overused or misused, can cause liver damage. Environmental toxins, such as certain chemicals, can also harm the liver.
- **Genetic Disorders**: Some people inherit conditions that can damage the liver, such as Wilson's disease or hemochromatosis.

4. How is liver disease diagnosed?

Liver disease is typically diagnosed through a combination of:

- **Blood Tests**: These can check for abnormal levels of liver enzymes or bilirubin, which can indicate liver damage.
- **Imaging**: An ultrasound or CT scan can provide a clear picture of the liver and detect any abnormalities such as fatty liver or tumors.
- **Liver Biopsy**: In some cases, a small sample of liver tissue may be taken to assess the degree of damage.
- **Endoscopy**: This procedure involves inserting a tube with a camera into the stomach to look for signs of liver disease-related complications, like varices.

5. What can I do to prevent liver disease?

Prevention of liver disease is primarily about making healthy lifestyle choices. Here are a few steps you can take to protect your liver:

- **Eat a healthy diet**: Focus on a balanced, nutrient-rich diet with lots of fruits, vegetables, whole grains, lean proteins, and healthy fats.
- **Limit alcohol consumption**: If you drink, do so in moderation, as excessive alcohol consumption is one of the leading causes of liver damage.
- **Exercise regularly**: Physical activity helps maintain a healthy weight, which can prevent liver diseases like fatty liver disease.
- **Get vaccinated**: Vaccines for hepatitis A and B can protect you from these viral infections that can damage the liver.
- **Avoid toxins**: Be mindful of exposure to harmful chemicals, and use medications only as prescribed by a doctor.

6. What is the role of diet in liver health?

Diet plays a crucial role in maintaining liver health. A liver-friendly diet can help reduce fat accumulation in the liver, prevent liver inflammation, and support detoxification. Foods that are particularly beneficial for liver health include:

- **Leafy Greens**: Spinach, kale, and other leafy vegetables help detoxify the liver.
- **Berries**: Rich in antioxidants, they help reduce liver inflammation.
- **Garlic**: Known to improve liver function by activating enzymes that help flush out toxins.
- **Olive Oil**: Contains healthy fats that support liver function and reduce fat buildup in the liver.
- **Turmeric**: Contains curcumin, a compound that has anti-inflammatory and liver-protective properties.

Conversely, it is best to avoid excessive consumption of fatty foods, processed sugars, and alcohol.

7. Can liver disease be reversed?

The potential for reversing liver disease depends on the stage and type of the condition. For example:

- **Fatty Liver Disease**: If caught early, this condition can often be reversed with lifestyle changes such as weight loss, exercise, and a healthy diet.
- **Hepatitis**: With appropriate antiviral treatment, some cases of hepatitis can be controlled, but chronic hepatitis can lead to long-term liver damage.
- **Cirrhosis**: While cirrhosis is generally not reversible, stopping the progression of the disease through lifestyle changes and medications can improve quality of life.

In general, early diagnosis and intervention are key to preventing further liver damage and improving liver function.

8. Is liver transplant the only option for severe liver disease?

Liver transplantation is typically considered when a person's liver has sustained irreversible damage and is no longer able to function. However, a transplant is a major surgery and is usually only recommended when other treatments have failed. Lifestyle changes, medications, and alternative therapies can help manage liver disease and potentially delay or prevent the need for a transplant.

9. What are the latest treatments for liver disease?

The field of liver disease treatment is constantly evolving. Some of the latest advancements include:

- **Gene Therapy**: Researchers are exploring gene therapy to treat genetic liver diseases like Wilson's disease and hemophilia.
- **Stem Cell Therapy**: Stem cells may be used in the future to regenerate liver tissue and help treat cirrhosis.
- **New Medications**: Recent breakthroughs in antiviral medications have significantly improved the treatment of hepatitis C.
- **Liver Regeneration**: Studies are being conducted on therapies that could help the liver regenerate itself more effectively.

It's important to stay up to date on the latest treatments, as new options are continuously becoming available.

Suggested Reading and Further Studies

1. "Liver Health" by Dr. Susan M. Smith

This book provides a deep dive into liver health, offering practical advice on how to support your liver through diet, exercise, and lifestyle changes. Dr. Smith, a leading expert in liver diseases, shares the latest research and medical recommendations for maintaining liver health and preventing liver disease.

2. "The Liver: A Complete Guide to Understanding the Liver and Liver Disease" by Dr. John G. Hunter

For those seeking a comprehensive guide to liver disease, this book covers everything from the basic anatomy and function of the liver to detailed explanations of liver diseases like hepatitis, cirrhosis, and fatty liver. It's perfect for readers who want a well-rounded understanding of liver health.

3. "Fatty Liver Disease: From Simple Fatty Liver to NASH and Cirrhosis" by Dr. Jeffrey S. Brown

This book focuses specifically on fatty liver disease, a condition that is becoming increasingly common in modern society. Dr. Brown breaks down the stages of fatty liver disease and offers actionable advice on how to manage and treat the condition with both conventional and alternative therapies.

4. "Healing the Liver Naturally" by Dr. Mark Hyman

Dr. Hyman is a well-known advocate for functional medicine, and in this book, he discusses the natural remedies and lifestyle changes that can support liver health. He emphasizes the importance of a clean diet, detoxification, and stress reduction for healing the liver.

5. Research Journals and Articles:

- **The Journal of Hepatology**: A peer-reviewed journal that publishes the latest research on liver diseases, treatments, and breakthroughs in the field.
- **Liver International**: This journal covers all aspects of liver disease, including pathophysiology, diagnostics, and therapeutic advancements.
- **Hepatology**: The official journal of the American Association for the Study of Liver Diseases, Hepatology is an essential resource for anyone looking to stay on top of the latest clinical research.

6. Online Resources:

- **American Liver Foundation (www.liverfoundation.org)**: This site offers a wealth of information on liver health, liver diseases, and the latest research findings.
- **Hepatitis B Foundation (www.hepb.org)**: A nonprofit organization dedicated to education, support, and research on hepatitis B.
- **National Institute of Diabetes and Digestive and Kidney Diseases (www.niddk.nih.gov)**: This government website provides valuable information on liver disease prevention, diagnosis, and treatment options.

7. Online Courses and Webinars:

- **Coursera - Liver Disease 101**: This free course provides an introduction to liver diseases and their treatments, ideal for those seeking to learn more at their own pace.
- **WebMD Liver Disease Webinar**: A series of webinars on liver health and the latest treatment options, presented by leading experts in the field.